about the authors

KATHY SNOWBALL, a former food director of *Australian Gourmet Traveller*, is a freelance food writer, menu and marketing consultant and educator. After a successful career in merchant banking, Kathy went to London to study at Leith's School of Food and Wine. Eight years of catering and teaching later, she returned home and joined the *Australian Women's Weekly* as assistant food editor. She then became part of the Gourmet Traveller team, becoming food editor in 1993 and food director in 2000. She has edited two cookbooks, *Gourmet Menus* and *Food for Friends*. Kathy also takes tours to the Sydney growers' markets, gives hands on cooking classes and is a partner in Manna from Heaven, bakers of divine handmade biscuits and cakes.

JAN PURSER is a naturopathic nutrition consultant, remedial therapist and meditation teacher. Jan's passion is teaching people how to become more balanced holistically through nutrition, diet, detoxification programs, counselling, meditation and natural therapies. Her busy clinic, Food, Body & Health, is based in Perth. Jan has worked in the food and food publishing industry for over 20 years and has been a practitioner since 1996. She is currently the contributing health editor to *Australian Good Taste* magazine and also writes for Weight Watchers magazine. Jan has written six books on health, food and meditation and her most recent books are *Indian Home Cooking* (with Ajoy Joshi) and *Blender Drinks* (with Dimitra Stais and Tracey Rutherford).

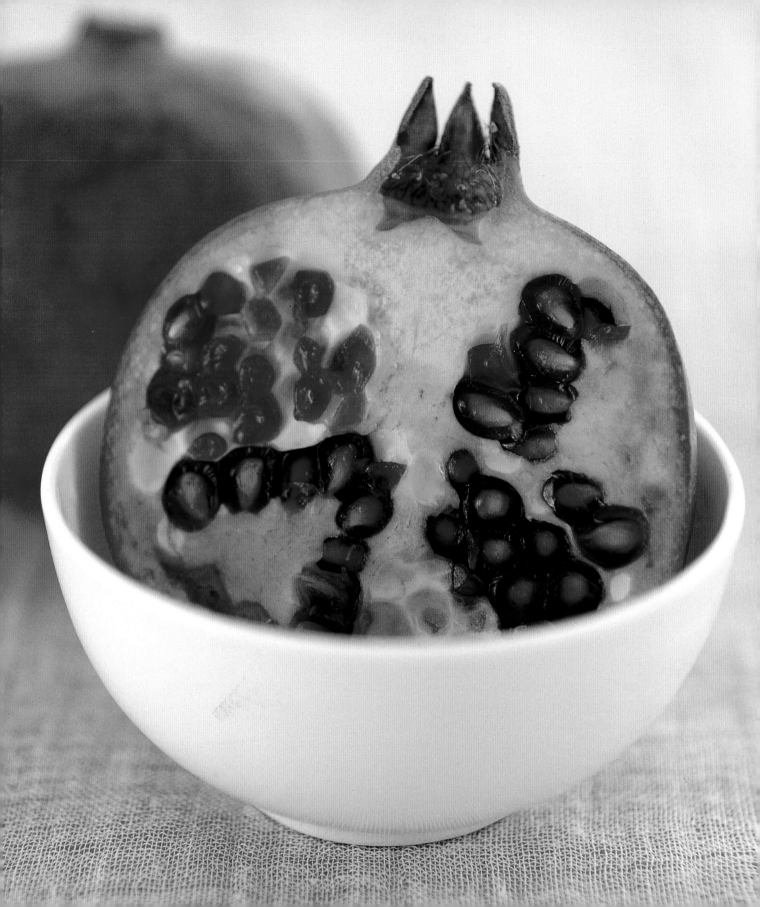

the
detox cookbook

CLEANSING FOR FOOD LOVERS

jan purser & kathy snowball

PHOTOGRAPHY BY GREG ELMS

A Sue Hines Book

Allen & Unwin

First published in 2004

A Sue Hines Book
Allen & Unwin Pty Ltd
83 Alexander Street
Crows Nest NSW 2065
Australia
Phone: (61 2) 8425 0100
Fax: (61 2) 9906 2218
Email: info@allenandunwin.com
Web: www.allenandunwin.com

National Library of Australia
Cataloguing-in-publication entry:
    Purser, Jan.
    The Detox Cookbook.
    ISBN 1 86508 969 9.
    1. Detoxification (Health). I. Snowball, Kathy. II. Title.
    III. Liver cleansing recipes
642.563

Photography by Greg Elms
Food styled by Virginia Dowzer
Typeset by Pauline Haas
Index by Fay Donlevy
Printed in China by Everbest
10 9 8 7 6 5 4 3 2

Our thanks to Minimax and Moss Melbourne for the generous loan of the dinnerware used in the photography, and to herb and vegetable growers Peter and Julie Cochrane.

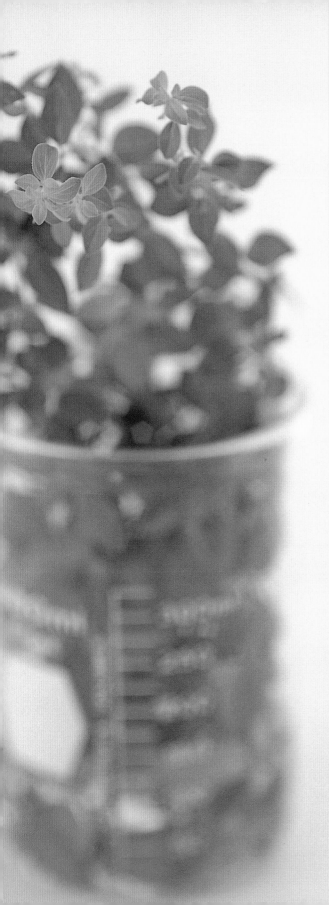

contents

about the book

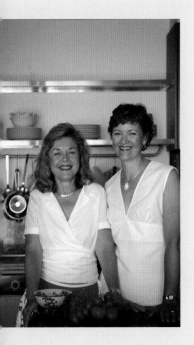

This book came about as result of a mutual love of good food and good health and a long and warm friendship.

While detoxing seems like a trendy subject, it has been the core therapy for most complementary medicine practitioners for decades. Naturopaths often begin their patient's treatment with a thorough detox to help reduce chronic symptoms and to begin the healing process.

Our detox program isn't a weight-loss 'diet', although if you follow our guidelines excess weight is bound to be shed without you even thinking about it. More importantly, it is a chance to give your body a rest from potential allergens and toxins so that it can regain balance, good health and vitality.

Many people believe healthy food is boring, but you don't have to sacrifice wonderful food when you are detoxing. That's what this book is all about. As foodies, we are not prepared to give up great tasting meals to be healthy so we came up with our own dishes that remain within the detox guidelines. The results astound our loved ones and friends, who don't realise they are eating detox food until they are told.

We want to share our philosophy of detoxing with you and to demystify some of the principles. We suggest you read through the first part of the book to gain an understanding of the why and how-to of detoxing. Following this, the recipe chapters are full of fabulous meals for every day and for entertaining. When you understand why detoxing works so well and realise how simple it can be, we are sure you will be converts. And when you taste our food, we know you won't be disappointed.

our stories

KATHY: About ten years ago I was complaining to Jan, my dear friend and health guru, that I was feeling run down, exhausted, puffy and bloated. In effect, I was having a moan about the pitfalls of working with food and wine. Jan immediately came forth with a solution as I knew she would – I needed to go on a detox. I was horrified at the idea – no wine (she must be joking), no caffeine (help), no wheat (how would I live without my daily intake of sourdough?), no dairy, no sugar... and so the list went on. What would I eat and drink? My life as a foodie would be over!

Under much duress, I eventually embarked on my first detox. Week one was a shocker. Headaches, feeling deprived, grumpy – to be honest, I was not a nice person to be around. However, by week two my energy levels were rising, I was sleeping like a baby and without any effort had lost a few kilos. I had planned to detox for a month, but I was feeling so good that I kept going for two.

Because I love food so much, I made a point of eating only the best produce. I developed new recipes that were within the boundaries so I didn't feel deprived. I now detox at least once, if not twice, a year for one to two months at a time. I see it as a regime (not a diet) that keeps me on track, maintains my energy levels and helps me shed weight that creeps on over the year. Now I look forward to my detox, knowing the benefits that come with it.

JAN: Some years ago, when I was in my mid twenties, I was experiencing poor health. I caught colds often and had other niggling and uncomfortable chronic symptoms such as persistent thrush and ear infections. After visiting a naturopath, I underwent a detox program, a little more strict than ours, for two months. I also took several supplements to help my body detoxify and re-balance.

The funny thing was that I started my first detox right at the beginning of working on a chocolate cookbook. I actually lost weight during that time, while many others I worked with gained a little. It was hugely challenging because chocolate is a major, major delight for me. However, the change in my health was remarkable and the results were really worth my efforts. My energy improved and all the annoying health problems disappeared. In fact, it was this experience that convinced me to study to become a natural therapist. Since that time, I have relished my yearly (or twice yearly) detox and my health has been mostly excellent. On the rare occasions I seem to catch a virus it's most likely because I'm working a bit too hard without taking some regular time out to recharge.

Detoxing can be such a foreign and daunting concept. I am extremely compassionate towards those starting a detox for the first time because I remember it well. I can only say how fabulous my clients feel after detoxing, and how quickly they adjust to the program. Many are reluctant to slip back into their old ways of eating and most come back for their yearly detox to keep their health in balance.

why detox?

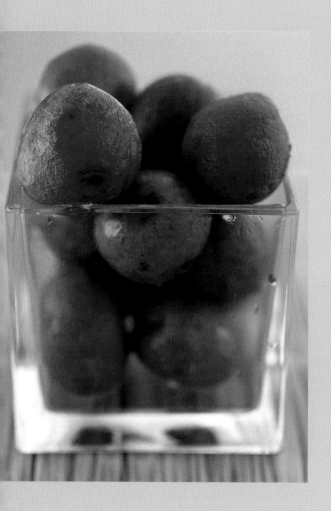

It's time to do a detox when you start finding it harder to get out of bed each morning, your waistline seems to have expanded beyond your waistband, you suffer with several colds a year, that skin rash is worsening, you reach for painkillers a little too often, you're suddenly taking antihistamine tablets for a chronic runny nose or hayfever, your tummy feels constantly bloated and you're producing a bit more gas than seems normal, the hormones take over each month turning you into an emotional or angry wreck, even small extra tasks seem like Mt Everest looming over you and you're reaching for caffeine and sugar as your daily close friends.

If this all sounds a bit too familiar, a detox will soon have you leaping out of bed ready to go for a walk, and the puffiness in your face and body will smooth over, leaving you looking younger and sparkling. In fact, you'll also most likely put away the antihistamines and painkillers, spend less on tissues, fit into your favourite clothes with ease, take on new projects with renewed enthusiasm, feel more motivated and positive, sleep more soundly, easily resist sugar and excess caffeine, and feel like your body is running like a well-oiled machine. It's remarkable the difference it makes, as many detox converts will heartily testify.

A detox does take a little organising, and you may feel a little worse rather than better over the first several days. However, once you're past the first patch, you won't look back. It's when your loved ones, friends and associates start asking you what you're doing to look so healthy and glowing that it really hits home how good you do feel – how easy it is to get through the day, and have energy left to burn.

do you need to detox?

Check the list of symptoms and lifestyle factors below. If you can tick two or more on either list, you would benefit greatly from our detox program. If you can tick lots, best plan that detox immediately!

SYMPTOMS

poor immunity (more than one cold or virus per year)

hayfever and other allergy symptoms

post-nasal drip (mucus running down back of throat)

chronic sore throat

headaches or migraines

puffiness under or around the eyes

dark shadows under the eyes

dry skin

pimples or acne

skin rashes such as eczema

abdominal bloating

poor digestion

heartburn or indigestion

constipation

regular diarrhoea

mucus in stools

excess flatulence or burping

chronic cystitis

tiredness on waking

excess fatigue

fluid retention in feet, legs and/or hands (puffiness, stiffness)

hormonal symptoms (PMS, menopausal, lumpy breasts)

chronic vaginal thrush or other irritations

muscle aches or pains

overreaction to situations

LIFESTYLE FACTORS

use of oral contraceptive pill or hormonal therapy

use of medications and prescribed drugs

use of antibiotics more than once in the past two years

exposure to chemicals (home, garden, pesticides, artificial food colourings and/or flavourings)

regular alcohol consumption (more than three drinks per week)

smoking or passive smoking

recreational drug use

regular exposure to traffic pollution

stressful lifestyle

two or more caffeine drinks daily (tea, coffee, cola, guarana, chocolate drinks)

excessive emotional stress

poor diet habits

eating takeaway food often

eating less than 5 serves of vegetables and 2 of fruit daily

eating deep-fried or fatty foods (more than once per fortnight)

the stress factor

When you are stressed your body creates hormones such as adrenaline and cortisol. Too much of these whipping around your system may lead to an increased risk of heart disease, hormone imbalance, poor immunity, high blood cholesterol and high blood pressure.

If you are tense or anxious much of the time due to busy work or family life, not to mention dealing with any emotional stress, your body will create toxins as by-products. Let's face it, life is demanding – how often can you say that you feel truly relaxed? A little stress *is* good for you as it gives you the drive to achieve the things you like to achieve. However, it is when you don't have a good balance of drive versus relaxation that you can feel overwhelmed and run into problems. A detox is the first step to turn your health around.

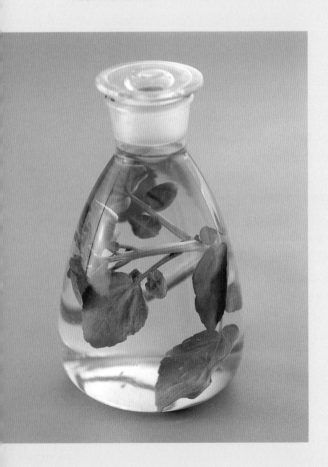

detox: the facts

WHAT ARE TOXINS?

Toxins are any substances, produced within your body or introduced into the body, that prevent the countless body processes maintaining optimum functioning. When toxins build up in your body, they affect every cell and the result is compromised health and possibly chronic disease.

As you go about your daily living, you are exposed to many toxins in the environment, both outdoors and within your home. Toxins from your environment, inhaled, ingested or absorbed through your skin, are called exotoxins. These include exhaust fumes; plastics; chemicals in cleaning products; chemicals used in building materials, furniture and furnishings; pesticides; herbicides; heavy metals; synthetic ingredients in cosmetics and other body products; oxidised fats in fried food; burnt fats in barbecued food; moulds; hormones given to some livestock; and food colours, preservatives and flavours. In fact, the complete list of environmental toxins you are regularly exposed to is overwhelming.

Endotoxins are toxins that form within the body. These toxins occur in several ways: if your digestive system isn't breaking down and assimilating food correctly; if you have what naturopaths call 'leaky gut syndrome', where larger than optimum food particles and waste matter are absorbed through damaged or inflamed intestinal membranes into the bloodstream and lymphatic system; if there is too little folic acid, vitamin B12 and B6 in your diet;

and/or if you are lacking dietary antioxidants (nutrients that prevent cell damage and deal with free radicals). In addition, you may introduce more toxins by choice, such as nicotine, alcohol, caffeine, overly processed foods and recreational drugs.

The result of all of this is an overloaded body that may not be able to keep up with the detoxification demands placed upon it. As the liver struggles to play its role in detoxification, some toxins recirculate through the body, essentially affecting most of the body systems by damaging cells and setting off inflammation which may eventually develop into chronic disease. When overload happens you are mostly likely to experience all kinds of niggly symptoms. Allergies, hayfever, hormonal imbalance, low energy, susceptibility to colds, fatigue, poor alcohol or caffeine tolerance, digestive disturbances and headaches are just a few initial complaints that may occur.

DETOXIFICATION IN THE BODY

Many chemical toxins are fat soluble and can settle in the body's fat cells if they are not eliminated. When this happens, it can be difficult to rid the body of these toxins unless fat loss occurs. If the toxins do settle in fat cells, they may contribute to symptoms of toxicity such as headaches, fatigue and muscle aches.

The liver plays a major role in the detoxification process in your body. It is a normal process that occurs every day of your life – although the efficiency of this depends on all the factors previously discussed. Naturopaths and other natural health practitioners have long held the view that to improve a patient's health, you must start by improving their liver function and digestion.

One role of the liver is to process and eliminate toxins that are delivered via the bloodstream (the liver filters up to two litres of blood per minute). Enzymes in the liver change the structure of toxic molecules, helping to reduce their toxicity and making them more water soluble. This is called Phase I detoxification: fat soluble toxins are converted into water soluble ones, making them easier to excrete.

In Phase II detoxification, enzymes attach the partially processed toxins to other molecules that assist in the toxins' elimination by making them even more water soluble and less toxic. The processed toxins are either directed to the kidneys to be excreted with the urine, or are added to bile in the gall bladder to end up in the intestinal tract and excreted (providing enough soluble fibre is present to absorb the toxins).

The two phases of detoxification occur quite rapidly and rely on the presence of particular amino acids, vitamins, minerals and other nutrients for smooth action. If there is a deficiency of any of these nutrients, the process may be impeded. If there is a load of toxins to be dealt with, and the liver is not functioning at its best, or is already overloaded, the process may not be completed properly. It is essential for both phases to work correctly for optimum detoxification to occur. If not, such as when the body is overloaded with toxins, the numbers of free radicals created during the process may cause cellular damage within the body, especially if there are inadequate supplies of antioxidants to prevent this damage. In addition, unprocessed toxins will recirculate in the body,

beginning the cycle once again, and adding even further to the overload.

Natural detoxification doesn't work efficiently when the body is overloaded, so you need to help your body eliminate toxins by consciously going on a detox program.

HOW A DETOX PROGRAM HELPS DETOXIFICATION

Our detox program works by eliminating from your diet foods and drinks that can create an extra burden on your liver (they may create toxins during their breakdown, or may be common allergens, such as wheat and dairy foods). The program also employs an array of fresh food along with specific additional nutrients to encourage efficient liver function, and incorporates soluble fibre into your daily diet to absorb toxins in the digestive tract to assist in their excretion. Once the toxic load is reduced, your liver has the opportunity to work more efficiently and it can get on with the business of detoxification. Toxins will be dealt with and eliminated and, bit-by-bit, your body will return to good balance, with annoying symptoms abating and your energy increasing.

We don't recommend strict fasts unless you are under the close supervision of a complementary health practitioner. Fasts that involve going without food or having greatly reduced food intake for days at a time may be too drastic for your body. Phase II detoxification requires particular nutrients such as amino acids to be efficient. Juice fasts or strict fasts don't supply these amino acids (found in proteins).

A gentle detox program such as ours can be sustained for a longer period of time, gaining greater long-term results, enabling you to go about your daily life with renewed energy. We find this a much preferable, and more sustainable, method of revitalising your body and health.

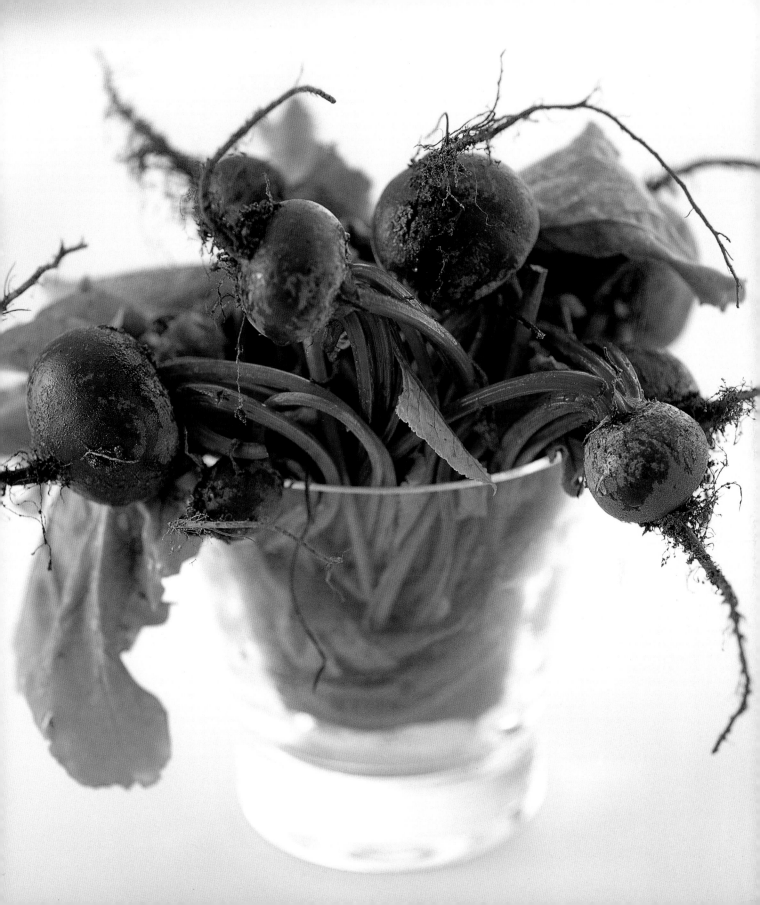

before you start

WHAT TO EXPECT

During the first few days of your detox you may have a headache or two due to caffeine withdrawal and from the actual detox process. It's also possible you may experience what seems like an unhappy digestive system for a few days until you settle into the detox. For this reason we strongly recommend you follow the advice under 'Extra fibre and supplements' (page 12) and 'Managing side effects' (page 9) to help reduce uncomfortable symptoms. Usually the first two to three days are the worst, then afterwards your energy will pick up and you'll begin to notice a difference in how you feel. As a general guide to reduce all symptoms, drink plenty of purified or spring water daily (see 'What to drink', page 11). During the first few days of detoxing, make sure you have time to rest if necessary. Following are some specific tips to managing a few possible symptoms.

WHEN TO START A DETOX

We always start our new year with a detox – it helps us to feel revived after the manic festive time where we all tend to eat, and perhaps drink, a little more than usual. It is an excellent way to enter a new year (and the ideal way to shed those festive kilos).

Consider starting your detox on a weekend where you have little planned. This way, if you do experience any discomfort such as the odd headache or fatigue, you can take it easy and even have a little nap if needed. Try to have few, if any, parties or other 'tricky' social events during the weeks you plan to detox.

Catered large functions can be difficult because you can't control what food is served. If any social events arise during your detox time, make sure you let your hosts know what foods you can't eat. In the case of catered parties, we suggest you have a good snack before you go in case the food isn't quite suitable. If you are dining out, it's quite easy to find items on most menus that are within the guidelines. See Lunch (page 45) and Dinner (page 95) for further hints and tips on this. It is quite possible to be socially active when you are detoxing and you can certainly have lots of fun. You will definitely have more energy for a great social life. Our fabulous recipes give you loads of options if you're entertaining at home.

PREPARING TO DETOX

We recommend that you gradually cut down your caffeine intake (tea, coffee, chocolate, cola, guarana drinks) over the week or so preceding your detox. This will help minimise caffeine withdrawal headaches in the first few days of your detox. You could also begin to increase the number of vegetables and legumes you eat to help your digestive system adjust to extra vegetable fibre.

It's always a good idea to do a good shop in preparation, purchasing the foods you will need during the first week of the program. See our 'Foods to eat' list on page 10 and choose some recipes you might start with to write your shopping list. And, read 'Extra fibre and supplements' on page 12 to add what you need to your list.

It's a great idea to let your family, friends and workmates know that you are starting a detox. This will help you socially – in fact, we find that most people are extremely interested to know what it involves and usually want to try it themselves, especially once they notice how sparky you look after a couple of weeks. If you are invited out it is best to warn your host you are not drinking alcohol and have a few dietary restrictions.

DURATION

We have both found that a four-week detox is a good length of time to achieve an excellent shift in wellbeing. Sometimes we detox for longer – six to eight weeks – and sometimes just for a week if we feel a bit sluggish and tired.

If you are planning your first detox, then stick with the program for at least four weeks to reap longer term benefits.

managing side effects

Headaches Take $\frac{1}{2}$ teaspoon of vitamin C powder in a glass of water twice a day. Have a snooze if possible. Rub a drop or two of lavender pure essential oil on your temples and neck. Dip a face cloth in chilled water, squeeze it out and place over your forehead. Take a homeopathic headache remedy (from health food stores).

Diarrhoea It's more likely that you may experience loose bowel movements rather than diarrhoea, and possibly more movements than usual. However, if you do have diarrhoea, drink lots of water, whisk 1 teaspoon of slippery elm powder, 1 teaspoon psyllium husks (excellent natural soluble fibre, from the health food store) and 1 teaspoon acidophilus bifidus powder (friendly bacteria, from the refrigerator in the health food store) into a glass of water and have 3 to 4 times a day. The symptoms usually don't persist beyond a day or two.

Flatulence Reduce the amount of legumes you eat if this is a problem. Chew your food slowly and don't drink fluids with your meals (many people feel more comfortable in their digestive system by following this advice). You may be reacting to extra vegetable fibre, in which case, eat lightly cooked vegetables until your body settles, then gradually increase the amount of raw vegetables you eat. If raw vegetables aren't commonplace in your diet, you may suffer with excess flatus. Sometimes fresh vegetable or fruit juices can create flatulence. In this case, make half the amount and dilute with an equal quantity of water.

Bloating Whisk 1 teaspoon acidophilus bifidus powder into a glass of water and have before each main meal. Some people feel bloated when they have psyllium husks. You can reduce the amount of psyllium you have by half or more. If you do this, increase the amount of freshly ground linseeds (from the health food store or supermarket) or slippery elm powder (excellent soluble fibre, from the health food store) you have (see 'Extra fibre and supplements' on page 12 – you need to have soluble fibre each day to absorb toxins in your digestive system). Don't overeat. Avoid too much soda water (the gas may exacerbate a bloated feeling).

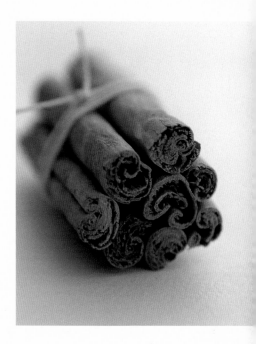

the detox program

We list here all the foods that will help support detoxification and will provide your body with wonderful antioxidants, vitamins and minerals. Some foods are common allergens and so we've put them on the list of foods to avoid. When these foods are ingested, they can add to the load on your liver and are best avoided during a detox for this reason. Some foods are okay in small amounts, but could be problematic in a larger quantity – we've listed these as the ones to limit. We have included a few foods that contain gluten in this list (rye, barley, spelt and oats), however, if you know that you are sensitive or allergic to gluten, please omit them entirely. If you're unsure of this, once you start your detox, take note of any digestive reactions you may have after eating these foods. If you do react, leave them out of your diet for the remainder of your detox.

FOODS TO EAT

Fresh vegetables lots of different coloured ones, both raw and cooked, preferably organic. If not, wash very well

Fresh fruit 2–3 pieces per day only, not melons or grapes, preferably organic

Legumes chickpeas, dried beans, lentils

Free-range poultry chicken, duck (without the fat), quail

Organic lamb and venison

Fish

Nuts and seeds (not peanuts)

Tofu, soy cheese, soy yoghurt choose those made from non-genetically modified soy beans (avoid these if you are sensitive to them)

Rice and rice products such as rice crispbread, noodles, pasta, puffed rice, crackers

Corn and corn products such as cornmeal/polenta and corn crispbread

Millet puffed and hulled

Quinoa (pronounced 'keen-wah') a grain that can be cooked like rice

Amaranth an 'ancient' nutritious grain

Buckwheat and buckwheat noodles check labels to ensure they are wheat free

Mung bean thread noodles

Gluten-free noodles and pasta

Gluten-free bread

Fresh vegetable juice and fruit juice see Juices (page 17)

Rice milk

Soy milk choose one made from non-genetically modified soy beans (avoid if you are sensitive to soy products)

Fresh herbs

Spices

Dried fish and bonito flakes

FOODS TO LIMIT

Free-range eggs try not to have more than 3 or 4 per week (avoid them altogether if you suffer with migraines or you suspect you are sensitive to them)

Dried fruit limit to 1 to 2 tablespoons per day (avoid any dried fruit that contains preservatives)

Olive oil, sunflower oil, canola oil

Butter use minimal butter

Vinegars use in dressings but don't overdo them (avoid these if you have had chronic thrush, tinea or cystitis – use lemon juice instead)

Mustard

Honey, maple syrup and rice syrup use sparingly as a sweetener in place of sugar

Miso use a small amount in soups, sauces and dressings

Naturally fermented soy and tamari sauces minimise or avoid these sauces if you have had recurring thrush, tinea, cystitis (avoid soy sauce if you have coeliac disease or if you are gluten or wheat sensitive)

Shellfish (avoid if you are allergic to or suspect you are sensitive to them)

Canned tomatoes okay on occasion, although fresh tomatoes are always preferable

Rye, spelt, barley and oat products bread, crispbread, muesli (avoid all these if you have coeliac disease or if you suspect you are sensitive to gluten)

FOODS TO AVOID

Wheat products pasta, noodles, bread, couscous, semolina, cakes, biscuits, pastry, wheat crispbread, savoury wheat biscuits, snack foods

Sugar and sugary foods white, brown and raw sugar, soft drinks, biscuits, cakes, slices, pastries, puddings, lollies, chocolate, 'health' bars, muesli bars

Artificial sweeteners

Alcohol all types

Caffeine tea, coffee, chocolate, cola, cocoa, guarana drinks or supplements

Dairy food milk, cream, sour cream, yoghurt, ice-cream, custard, creamy sauces, cheese, dried milk

Yeast and fermented products bread, yeast extract spreads, beer, wine, fermented fish and oyster sauces, soy sauce (see Foods to limit) – wheat-free tamari sauce is okay

Canned vegetables

Oranges and orange juice especially if you suffer with migraines

Colourings, flavourings, preservatives and chemical or articial additives

Soft drinks soda water and plain mineral water are okay

Melons and grapes these are high in fruit sugar

Dried fruit containing preservatives check labels on packets

Processed meats or poultry, salami, bacon, ham these contain preservatives and other additives

Peanuts and peanut butter a common allergen, may be contaminated by aflatoxins (toxins produced by a mould that grows on peanuts)

Peanut oil

Beef, pork or veal organic varieties are okay limited to one serve per week

Deep-fried or shallow-fried food

Concentrated tomato products canned tomato puree or paste, tomato sauce, bottled or canned tomato-based pasta sauces

Fatty food

Any foods you are allergic to or suspect you are sensitive to

WHAT TO DRINK

It is very important to drink enough liquid during each day to help your body flush out toxins. You need to drink at least 2 litres (8 cups) of liquid a day and this can be in the form of any or all of the options below. Diluted or undiluted freshly extracted juices (see Juices, page 17) also contribute to your liquid intake, but for these purposes are really considered a 'food' rather than a plain liquid because they contain such concentrated nutrients.

Purified and spring water

Soda water with a squeeze of fresh lemon or lime juice

Herbal tea avoid flavoured black or green teas

Hot water with slices of fresh ginger and/or lemon

Dandelion root coffee

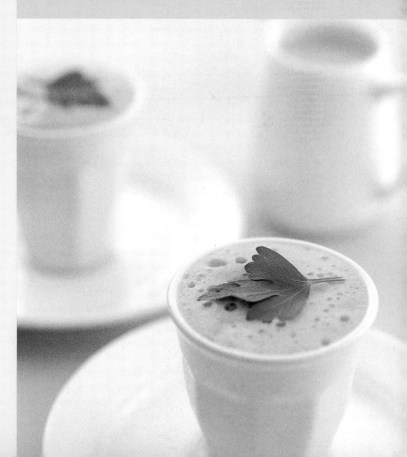

extra fibre & supplements

FIBRE

Fibre is essential in your daily diet to help absorb and eliminate toxins from your digestive system. Choose from the options below and have two serves per day, at breakfast and later in the day (afternoon tea is a good time to reduce sugar cravings and help reduce appetite).

1 tbsp freshly ground linseeds (4.5g dietary fibre) sprinkle over cereal, add to a smoothie, stir into a soup, whisk into fresh juice, mix into soy yoghurt or chopped fruit

1$^{1}/_{2}$ tsp psyllium husks (2.8g dietary fibre) whisk into a glass of water, juice or smoothie and drink immediately (psyllium absorbs liquid quite quickly, so drink lots of water afterwards)

2 tsp pure slippery elm bark powder (2.1g dietary fibre) whisk into a glass of water, juice or smoothie and drink immediately (it will thicken the liquid quite quickly)

1 tbsp oat bran (1.4g dietary fibre) **or rice bran** (2.3g dietary fibre) sprinkle over cereal, add to a smoothie, stir into a soup, mix into soy yoghurt or chopped fruit

SUPPLEMENTS

Some nutrients and herbs assist your liver and digestive system to function at their best and in turn assist your body to detoxify. These are not compulsory but will improve the overall benefits.

Antioxidant complex Antioxidants help prevent damage caused by free radicals in your body. The complex should contain nutrients such as vitamins C, E and A (or betacarotene) and B vitamins. A good supplement may also contain antioxidants such as grape seed extract, St Mary's thistle (milk thistle) and/or selenium. Have 1 or 2 tablets per day with meals (check dosage on the label).

Acidophilus and bifidus powder This will help ensure your digestive system is well stocked with 'friendly' bacteria to assist with optimum digestion. Take $^{1}/_{2}$ teaspoon of powder two times per day, mixed into a glass of water (you can mix it with your fibre option) and drink just before meals.

Liver formula This will help your liver function at its best, aiding detoxification and digestion. A good formula may contain nutrients such as DL-methionine, choline bitartrate, inositol, L-glutamine, B6 and/or dandelion (*Taraxacum officinale*) and artichoke (*Cynara scolymus*). Take 1 tablet two to three times per day with meals (check dosage on the label).

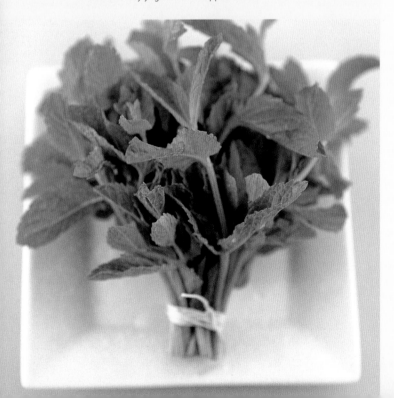

the program food plan

This is a guide on what to eat at each meal to ensure you are eating a good mix of nutrients.
This will help you to sustain good energy.

BREAKFAST

Freshly made juice (see Juices, page 17). You may prefer to have your juice later in the day, say, before dinner. Have only 1 undiluted juice or 2 diluted juices per day.

Protein egg, nuts and seeds, fish, chicken, tofu, meat, legumes, soy cheese, soy yoghurt (this supplies a little protein along with carbohydrate). Include a small portion of protein with your breakfast (60–80g).

Carbohydrate gluten-free bread or rye bread, cooked rice, rice or corn crispbread, soy or rice milk, puffed rice or millet, rolled oats or rice, gluten-free muesli (our recipe on page 27 contains protein and carbohydrate), cooked potato, soy yoghurt, gluten-free pancakes. Have $1/2$ to 1 cup of carbohydrate.

Fruit and/or vegetables most of our breakfast recipes include a fresh fruit or vegetable or two. You can save fruit for between meal snacks if you prefer.

Extra fibre and supplements see page 12. Include these with *every* breakfast.

LUNCH

Protein in addition to the breakfast protein list, choose from venison, duck, quail, lamb and shellfish. Have a portion of a protein food to suit your appetite.

Carbohydrate in addition to the breakfast list, choose from rice noodles, buckwheat noodles, cooked buckwheat, quinoa, amaranth and polenta. Have 1 to 2 slices of bread, 2 to 4 crispbread, or the equivalent of $1/2$ to 1 cup cooked carbohydrate.

Vegetables, raw and/or cooked Have the equivalent of 2 to 3 cups of vegetables, preferably of different colours. You can choose from one of our gorgeous salad recipes in Basics (see page 158) if you like.

Fruit

DINNER

Protein as for breakfast and lunch. Have a portion of a protein food to suit your appetite.

Carbohydrate as for breakfast and lunch. Have the equivalent of $1/2$ to $3/4$ cup.

Vegetables as for lunch. Have 3 to 4 cups of different coloured vegetables.

Extra fibre and supplements see page 12. You may prefer to have these at afternoon tea time.

Fruit You may like to finish your meal with a piece of fruit, or choose one of our dessert recipes.

SNACKS

Choose from one of our snack recipes in Snacks, page 33. Or have one of the following:

Fruit one piece or two

Unsalted nuts and/or seeds a small handful

Corn or rice crispbread spread with Hummus (page 165) or Almond and Seed Spread (page 38) or soy cheese

Soy yoghurt a small container (You can mix this with fruit and/or nuts and seeds, plus your fibre option.)

lifestyle

EXERCISE

If you already exercise regularly, keep up your routine, although you may like to slow down a little during the first few days of your detox. If you don't exercise regularly, the end of week one of your detox is a good time to start going for a daily walk. Exercise helps your body to function well and is extremely important for overall health and emotional wellbeing. Walking is the easiest of all exercise to manage and you could start with 15 minutes per day if you are unfit, gradually building up to 45 minutes of brisk walking per day. Include some hills as your fitness improves.

Exercise aids digestive function, helps reduce constipation, reduces stress, helps with muscle tone, helps maintain a healthy weight and decreases cardiovascular disease risk. One of the benefits that is particularly helpful for detoxing is increased circulation – both blood circulation and lymphatic flow. This helps reduce fluid retention and encourages the lymphatic system to move toxins through the body to be eliminated.

MIND DETOX

This is a great time to detox your mind while you detox your body. Consider doing a meditation course or listening to relaxation or meditation CDs or tapes during your detox (available from good book stores). The benefits of meditation are excellent – reduced blood pressure, improved sleep, better concentration, improved creativity and productivity, more motivation, less negative self-talk, and a more relaxed outlook.

Spend 10 to 15 minutes per day in meditation. You can simply sit quietly concentrating on your breathing and allowing your thoughts to come and go.

You could also spend time during your detox to reflect on your beliefs and attitudes. This is a good time to clear out those that don't serve you well and replace them with a fresh view. Ask yourself if you make choices based on fear or courage. If your choices are based on fear, you are most likely creating toxins in your body. When your choices are based on courage, your body naturally creates the hormones that help you to feel happy and uplifted.

Ask yourself if you are holding onto resentment, anger, guilt, shame or blame. These emotions are toxic to your soul and drain away your precious life energy. This drain is thought to eventually manifest in your body as physical symptoms or disease, or as depression. Hold the intention to resolve old issues, seeking professional help if needed, so that you can redirect your energy into fulfilling and joyful pursuits. Unresolved issues from your past can hold you back from growing as a person as every choice you make, and your attitude to your life, are affected deeply by them. Resolve to forgive yourself and others for choices and hurts gone by. Your health – emotional and physical – will improve dramatically when you live each day with optimism, courage, trust, faith and joy.

LIFESTYLE FACTORS TO AVOID

Naturally, if you are about to do a detox program, you might have to reduce or avoid some of the 'extras'.

Alcohol Avoid all types of alcohol.

Nicotine If it's possible to cut down or avoid altogether, your body will find it even easier to get into detox mode. If you think you can't cut down, then do a detox regardless because it will still help your body deal with the toxins.

Recreational drugs We suggest you give them a break while you detox.

Chemicals If you work with paints or other products that contain chemicals, you would benefit greatly from a regular detox. In this case, it may be simply too hard to avoid chemicals. Definitely detox, rather than not, and make sure you follow the advice in the Extra Fibre and Supplements section so that your body has all the support it needs. Wear a mask when dealing with chemicals, such as paints, pesticide sprays, herbicide sprays and other chemical-based products. This is important if you suffer with asthma or allergic reactions that affect your sinuses or breathing.

Barbecues We suggest that you barbecue on a hotplate rather than an open grill over charcoals. Reason being that fats dripping onto the coals, along with the high cooking temperatures, can create carcinogenic compounds on the food. Avoid overbrowning food. Marinating the food helps reduce the risk of these compounds forming.

Stress Take the time during your detox to minimise stress. This is an important part of the detox – it will help your body get on with the job, rather than keeping on 'high alert'. Get to bed a bit earlier, avoid working excessive hours and take regular time out to relax. Spend time with friends and family – and laugh a lot (an excellent tonic).

maintaining the balance

POST DETOX

To retain the benefits of your detox, very gradually re-introduce foods to your diet. After your first detox we suggest you keep a food diary for a fortnight or so to record reactions to foods or drinks. Begin by re-introducing single foods to your diet so that you can monitor any reactions. This is especially useful if you have been suffering with chronic symptoms or low energy – you may discover what was causing any niggling symptoms before you began your detox. In this case, try to limit the offending food or drink in your diet to minimise ongoing symptoms – you may be able to tolerate the food just once or twice per week.

Try not to go immediately back to your usual way of eating and drinking. Continue having a fresh vegetable juice each day and have four to five alcohol free days for a couple of weeks or so. Treat your body kindly to keep the detox benefits going longer term. This will improve not only your physical, but also your emotional, wellbeing.

DETOX TOP UPS

To keep a feeling of ongoing balance and good health in your body and mind, consider doing a detox yearly or twice yearly. It is an excellent way to help keep your immunity up to speed and to manage your weight effectively.

If you like, you can do a 'mini' detox from time to time – following the regime for just two to three days. We often follow our detox guidelines on weekdays to keep our bodies in balance during very busy working or social periods.

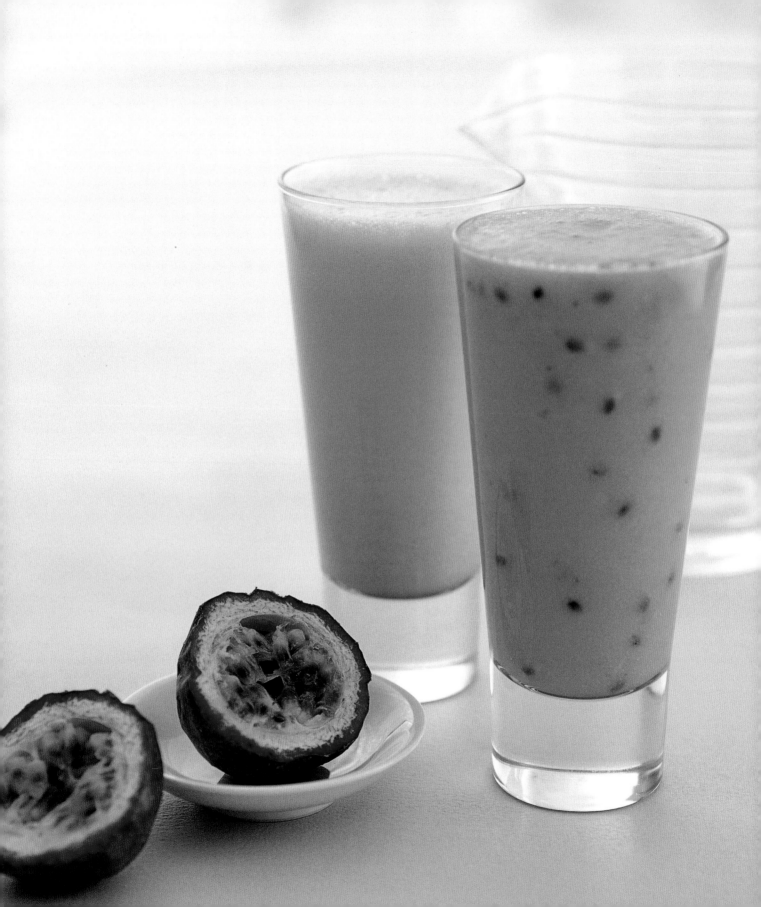

juices

Have a glass of warm water with half a fresh lemon squeezed into it first thing in the morning to kick-start your digestive system.

Fresh vegetable and fruit juices contain a wonderful array of live enzymes and substances called phytochemicals which act as anti-oxidants in your body. You will gain excellent benefits from one to two juices a day. You can dilute the juices with purified or spring water, or soda water to make them lighter if you prefer.

Choose from our selection depending on your needs of the day. For example, we'd recommend you try to have a detox support juice just about every day. If your digestion has been a bit tricky of late, try the digestion aid juice with your main meal. We think of the tropical breakfast juice as a good one for that leisurely weekend breakfast. And if you have problems with body odour or skin problems, have the clean green juice on a regular basis.

If you like, you can whisk 1 teaspoon of psyllium husks or slippery elm powder into your glass of juice to boost your soluble fibre intake (see page 12). This will assist detoxification by absorbing toxins in your digestive system and helping to prevent their reabsorption into your body.

KATHY: My favourite juice is the detox support juice and I love to have it about 6.30 pm when I am preparing dinner. Apart from the fact that it tastes fabulous and you can feel it doing you good, it is also very filling and I find that it really takes the edge off my appetite at that tricky time of day when it could be so easy to pick at food before dinner.

JAN: I like to start my day with the detox support juice. I can feel the goodness surging through my body and I find it helps with regularity, especially with the addition of some fibre (see Extra Fibre & Supplements, page 12). The fibre also helps slow down the digestion of breakfast, helping to sustain good energy throughout the morning.

detox support juice

The beetroot in this juice will help your liver play its role in detoxification. You can have this juice as part of breakfast, between meals or as a pre-dinner drink. You can add your extra fibre option to this juice if you like. If you suffer from gout, take the leaves off the celery.

4 large carrots

4 sticks celery, leaves attached

1/2 scrubbed beetroot

6 sprigs fresh parsley, stems attached

4 cm piece ginger

Cut vegetables into pieces large enough to fit into feed tube of your juice extractor. Process vegetables, parsley and ginger and pour into a jug. Mix well and drink immediately.

SERVES 2

digestion aid juice

This is a great juice to have to assist with digestion. The natural enzymes in pineapple help to break down the protein food you eat. This also makes a lively summer drink – add ice cubes and a dash of soda water.

1 ripe pineapple, peeled

4 cm piece ginger

1/4 cup fresh mint leaves

Cut pineapple into pieces that will fit in the feed tube of your juice extractor. Process pineapple, ginger and mint and pour into a jug. Mix well. Drink immediately.

SERVES 2

clean green juice

The chlorophyll in green vegetables is thought to help with the detoxification processes. In addition, chlorophyll is useful in treating smelly feet, bad breath and body odour. This is a light refreshing juice that makes you feel clean from the inside out. Add ice cubes if you like.

2 Lebanese (small green) cucumbers
1/2 green capsicum, seeded
6 sprigs fresh parsley, stems attached
2 green apples, quartered and cored

Cut vegetables and apples into pieces that will fit in feed tube of your juice extractor. Process vegetables, parsley and apples and pour into a jug. Mix well and drink immediately.

SERVES 2

tropical breakfast juice

This is a lovely juice to have while the tropical fruit is in season. You can use pawpaw or papaya, depending on which is available. If you like, add the juice of a lime for extra zing.

1/2 ripe pineapple, peeled
500 g pawpaw, seeded
1 small or 1/2 large banana
pulp from 2 passionfruit

Cut pineapple and pawpaw into pieces that will fit in the feed tube of your juice extractor. Process pineapple and pawpaw and pour into a blender jug. Add banana and blend until well combined, then stir in passionfruit pulp and drink immediately.

SERVES 2

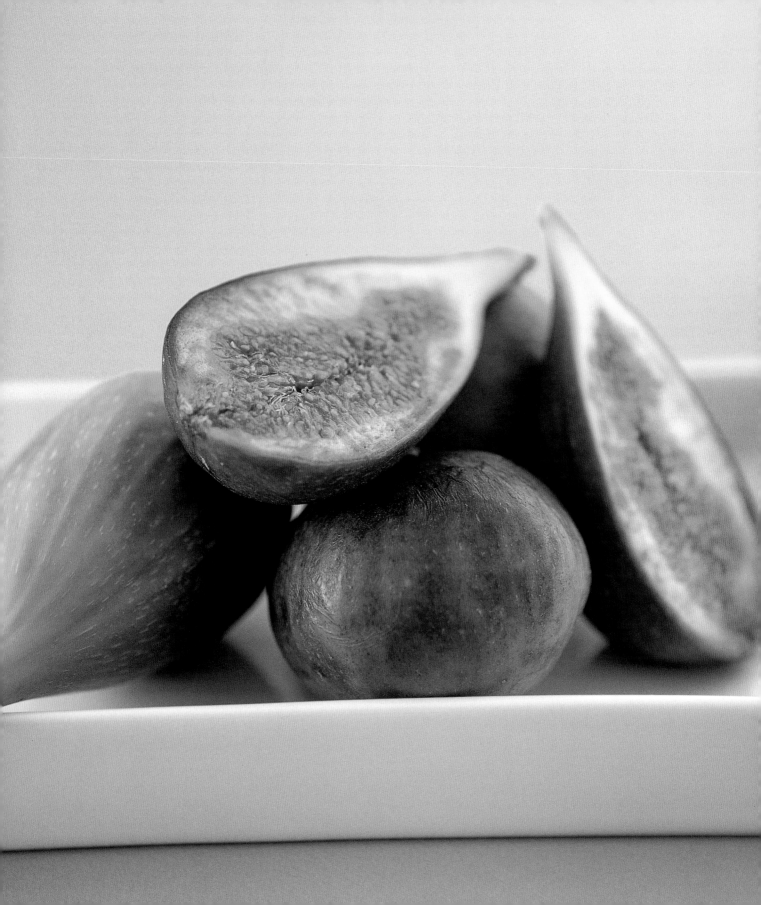

breakfast

KATHY: I am definitely not a breakfast person and only eat it under sufferance. I am not really interested in serious food until about 12 pm, and then I am looking for something savoury. Over the years Jan has persuaded me to eat a healthy breakfast to see me through the morning and I do see the logic. However I still prefer something light such as fruit and a handful of almonds, or if I am really lashing out I will have a bowl of gluten-free muesli like the recipe on page 27. That's about it for me!

JAN: Breakfast is an important meal for me and I like to eat a combination of protein and carbohydrates because I find that mixture takes me through the morning well. Eating out for breakfast is a favourite weekend treat for my partner Gavin and I, and I usually order poached eggs, mushrooms and spinach or bok choy when detoxing. I'll also ask for a fresh vegetable juice and drink peppermint tea instead of coffee or regular tea.

You may be a big hearty breakfast person, or you may be an 'I can only stomach fruit in the morning' person. Whichever the case, make sure you do have breakfast as it is an important meal. Ideally, you would have some kind of protein (see page 13) along with some carbohydrate and a little fat. However, if fruit is your thing, then keep it simple. Add some nuts as well, maybe a little later in the morning. You may even enjoy our smoothie which is quite light, but provides a good range of nutrients.

If you suffer migraines, you might prefer to avoid dishes containing eggs as these may be a trigger for you. For all others, don't have more than 3 to 4 eggs per week during your detox.

If you are having breakfast out, try your best to choose dishes that are within our guidelines. Some good choices are muesli with soy milk and fruit, poached eggs with mushrooms and spinach, fruit salad with soy yoghurt or a soy and fruit smoothie.

super smoothie

If you're in a hurry for breakfast, this is a great option because it's so easy to throw together. The combination of fruit, linseeds and almonds will give you good energy through the morning. If you like, you can add $1/2$ teaspoon psyllium husks or $1^1/2$ teaspoons oat bran for extra soluble fibre.

250 ml (1 cup) rice milk or soy milk

1 small or $1/2$ large ripe banana, quartered

$1/2$ cup fresh or frozen blueberries

1–2 tbsp linseeds, freshly ground

1–2 tbsp almond meal

1 tsp honey, rice syrup or maple syrup

Place all the ingredients in a blender jug and blend until thick and smooth. Pour into a glass and drink immediately.

SERVES 1

Best made just before drinking as it will thicken on standing.

gluten-free flat bread
with spread & avocado

Based on traditional Indian flat bread, this bread is easy to make and will keep well in the freezer so that you can simply pop one in the toaster to warm through. The combination of bread with the Almond & Seed Spread makes a fair source of protein and will give you good energy for the morning. We also like this bread topped with Hummus (page 165), avocado and beetroot.

300 g (2 cups) all-purpose gluten-free
    flour mix
2 tsp gluten-free baking powder
canola or light olive oil
Almond & Seed Spread (page 38)
ripe avocado, seeded, peeled and sliced

Sift flour mix and baking powder into a bowl and make a well in centre. Add 1 tablespoon of oil and about 180 ml (3/4 cup) water. Use a round-bladed knife in a cutting motion to mix ingredients. Use your hand to bring mixture together into a firm dough. Knead in bowl until smooth. Divide dough evenly into 8 portions. Shape each portion into an oval and roll out on very lightly floured surface to an oval about 13 cm in length.

Heat a large heavy-based frying pan over medium-high. Brush one side of flat bread lightly with oil and place, oil-side down, in pan. Cook for 3 minutes or until lightly browned underneath. Brush surface lightly with oil. Turn and cook other side, pressing edges with a clean cloth occasionally, for 2 minutes or until lightly browned. Cool on wire rack. Repeat cooking with remaining flat bread.

To serve, spread bread with Almond & Seed Spread and top with the avocado slices.

MAKES 8 FLAT BREAD

Place cooled bread into a sealed freezer bag and freeze for up to 1 month. Wrap in foil and warm in oven at 150°C for 10–15 minutes, or pop into a toaster to thaw and heat through.

poached eggs with wilted bok choy & garlic mushrooms

This breakfast will see you through the morning very nicely. The nutrition it supplies is excellent – great anti-oxidants from the greens with fibre from the mushrooms and, of course, good quality protein and a whole range of nutrients from the eggs. Poach the eggs just before serving. You can serve the mushrooms at room temperature if you like, with toasted rye bread or gluten-free bread.

2 tsp olive oil

1 large clove garlic, finely chopped

250 g Swiss brown mushrooms, sliced

2 tbsp finely chopped fresh flat-leaf parsley

2 tbsp white vinegar

4 large eggs

1 bunch baby bok choy, quartered lengthways

3 tsp wheat-free tamari sauce

freshly ground black pepper

Heat oil in a small frying pan over medium heat. Cook garlic and mushrooms in pan, stirring occasionally, for 4 minutes or until soft. Stir in parsley and season to taste. Remove from heat and cover to keep warm.

Bring a deep frying pan of salted water to the boil, add the vinegar, then reduce to a gentle simmer. Carefully break 1 egg into a small bowl. Use a wooden spoon to swirl the water in pan to create a whirlpool. Tip egg into centre of whirlpool and cook for 4 minutes or until set on the outside. Use a slotted spoon to lift onto a plate lined with paper towel. Continue cooking eggs, placing on the plate when done.

Meanwhile, cook bok choy in top half of a steamer over boiling water for 4–5 minutes or until just tender. Remove from heat.

Carefully lift eggs from plate and return to frying pan of hot water to heat for 1 minute. Lift onto paper towel to drain quickly then place on serving plates. Place mushrooms and bok choy on plates, drizzling bok choy with tamari. Sprinkle with black pepper and serve immediately.

SERVES 2–3

Best made just before serving

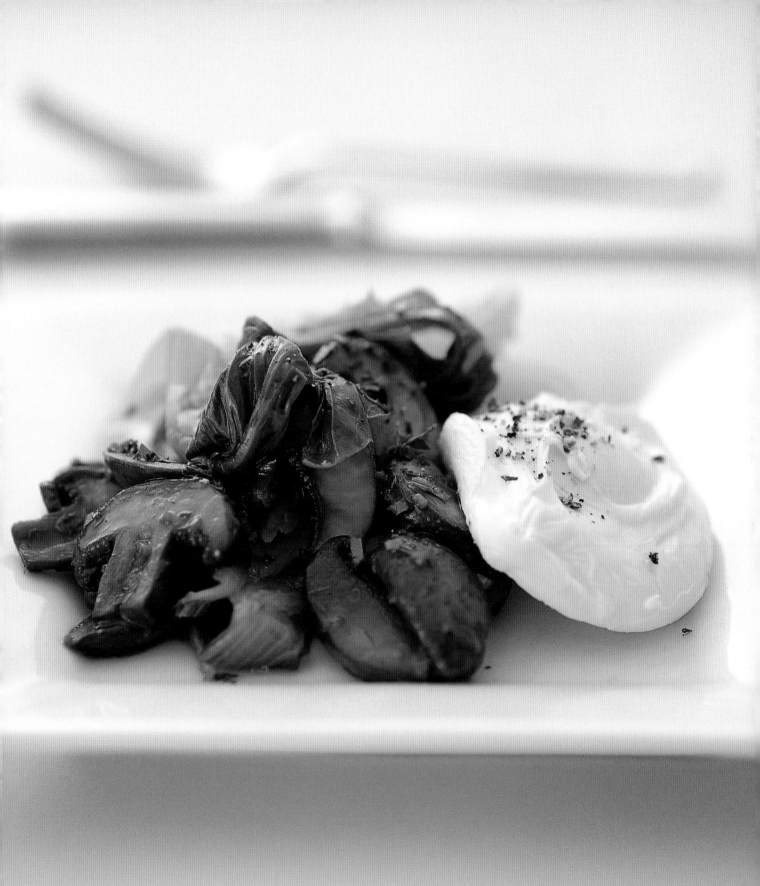

free-range egg omelette with herbs

The trick is not to overcook the omelette – leave the top just a little soft before folding it and serving. This makes a wholesome breakfast dish, or light meal. Serve with toast if you like.

5 eggs

3 green (spring) onions, trimmed and finely chopped

2 tbsp chopped fresh chives

2 tbsp chopped fresh flat-leaf parsley

2 tbsp chopped fresh coriander

1 tbsp chopped fresh oregano

2 tsp butter

Whisk eggs and 2 tablespoons water in a bowl. Add green onions and herbs and season to taste.

Melt butter in an omelette pan over medium heat. Pour in egg mixture and cook for 4–5 minutes or until almost set on top. Fold omelette in half, cut in half crossways and serve hot.

SERVES 2

Best made just before serving

gluten-free muesli

Make sure you buy preservative-free dried fruit. You can substitute any of the dried fruit with your favourites, depending on what you have available. We prefer the smaller paler puffed rice as they have lots of crunch to offer. We like to eat this with soy or rice milk and some fresh berries scattered on top. You can also add a good dollop of soy yoghurt if you like, along with your fibre option (see page 12). To make a larger quantity, you can just double or triple the recipe.

50 g (1/2 cup) flaked almonds

25 g (1/3 cup) shredded coconut

110 g (2 cups) puffed rice

30 g (2 cups) puffed millet

115 g (1 cup) rice bran

80 g (1/2 cup) pumpkin seed kernels

55 g (1/3 cup) dried currants

35 g (1/4 cup) thinly sliced dried apricots

10 g (1 1/3 cup) chopped dried apples

Spread almonds on oven tray and bake at 180°C for 5 minutes or until lightly toasted. Cool.

Spread coconut on oven tray and cook in oven for 3 minutes or until lightly toasted. Cool.

Combine almonds and coconut with remaining ingredients in a large bowl. Mix well. Transfer to an airtight container.

MAKES ABOUT 7 1/4 CUPS OR 8 SERVES

Muesli will keep for 6 weeks in airtight container in a cool cupboard.

dill rice patties with smoked salmon & cucumber dressing

This is a very smart looking breakfast that is easy to make. You can use a 60 ml (^{1}/4 cup) measure to make 8 patties to serve 4 if you like. You can also serve this dish as a light meal with a salad.

150 g (^{2}/3 cup) medium-grain rice,
   cooked

2 eggs

3 green (spring) onions, finely chopped

2 tbsp chopped fresh dill

grated rind 1 lemon

2 tsp olive oil

100 g smoked salmon, cut into strips

Fresh dill sprigs to serve

CUCUMBER DRESSING

1 Lebanese (small green) cucumber,
   diced

175 g (^{3}/4 cup) plain soy yoghurt

2 tbsp chopped fresh dill

1 tbsp lemon juice

Combine rice, egg, green onions, dill and lemon rind in a bowl and mix well. Season to taste. Heat olive oil in a large non-stick frying pan over medium heat. Pack rice mixture into an 80 ml (^{1}/3 cup) measure then tip into pan and flatten mixture slightly into a patty shape. Place 2 more patties in pan. Cook for 3 minutes or until lightly browned underneath, then use an egg lifter to carefully turn patties. Cook for a further 3 minutes or until lightly browned. Place on a plate and cover to keep warm. Repeat with remaining mixture to make a total of 6 patties.

To make Cucumber Dressing, combine all ingredients in a bowl and season to taste.

Place patties on serving plates, top with salmon and spoon dressing over the top. Garnish with dill sprigs.

SERVES 3
MAKES 6 PATTIES

Patty mixture can be made a day ahead. Keep, covered, in refrigerator. Bring to room temperature before cooking and cook just before serving.

Dressing is best made on day of serving.

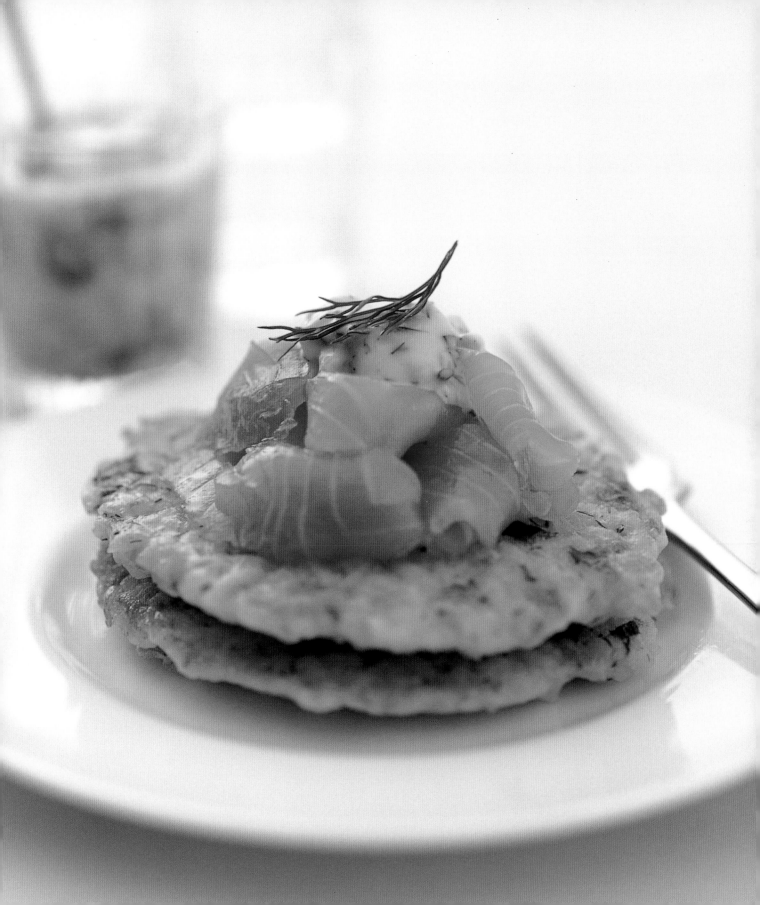

rice congee

Congee is the ultimate Asian comfort food. It is an excellent dish to eat when you don't feel very well because it is so nurturing. As a breakfast meal (or at any other time of day), it provides good nutrition.

1.5 L (6 cups) Chicken or Vegetable Stock (page 159)

100 g ($^1/_2$ cup) medium-grain rice

200 g organic chicken breast or boneless white fish fillet or firm tofu, diced

1 tbsp grated ginger

1$^1/_2$ tsp sesame oil

4 green (spring) onions, thinly sliced

$^1/_4$ cup chopped fresh coriander

40 g ($^1/_4$ cup) slivered almonds, toasted

1 small red chilli, thinly sliced

1 tbsp packaged fried onions

Bring stock to the boil in a saucepan. Add rice and simmer, partially covered, for 1$^1/_2$ hours or until a runny porridge consistency. Combine chicken, fish or tofu with ginger and sesame oil in a bowl. Add to rice mixture and cook about 5 minutes or until chicken or fish is cooked through. Season to taste.

Ladle into bowls and sprinkle with green onions, coriander, almonds, chilli and fried onion. Serve hot.

SERVES 4

The congee mixture can be made a day or two ahead and reheated for breakfast. You may need to add a little extra stock to soften the consistency – it should be like a runny porridge. Keep in an airtight container in the refrigerator. Add the green onions, almonds, chilli and fried onions just before serving.

buckwheat pancakes with cinnamon apples & maple syrup

The pancakes are light and fluffy and are best made close to serving. This is a delicious breakfast for those who enjoy pancakes. The cinnamon apples make a sweet and saucy accompaniment without weighing you down with sugar.

110 g (¾ cup) all-purpose gluten-free
　flour mix

110 g (¾ cup) buckwheat flour

3 tsp gluten-free baking powder

250 ml (1 cup) rice milk

2 eggs

2 tsp pure maple syrup

melted butter, for greasing

CINNAMON APPLES

5 red apples, quartered, cored and
　peeled

1 tbsp pure maple syrup

½ tsp ground cinnamon

Sift flour mix, buckwheat flour and baking powder into bowl. Make well in centre. Whisk together rice milk, eggs and maple syrup. Gradually stir into flour mixture and whisk to a smooth batter. Set aside for 15 minutes.

To make Cinnamon Apples, cut apple quarters in halves lengthways. Place in saucepan with 180 ml (¾ cup) water, maple syrup and cinnamon. Bring to the boil, then reduce heat to medium-low and cook, covered, for 15 minutes or until apples are tender. Remove half the apple pieces to a bowl. Use hand blender to puree remaining apples in pan or mash with potato masher. Return apple pieces and stir through.

Use folded piece kitchen paper to grease a large non-stick frying pan with melted butter very lightly and heat over medium heat. Place two to three 60 ml (¼ cup) lots of pancake batter in pan and cook for 1–2 minutes or until bubbles appear on surface and pancakes are golden underneath. Turn pancakes and cook other side until golden. Transfer to a plate and cover with a clean cloth to keep warm. Repeat with remaining batter to make 12 pancakes.

Serve warm pancakes topped with warm Cinnamon Apples.

SERVES 4–6

Batter can be made several hours ahead and kept, covered, at room temperature. You can make the cinnamon apples a day ahead. Keep covered in the refrigerator. Warm through to serve.

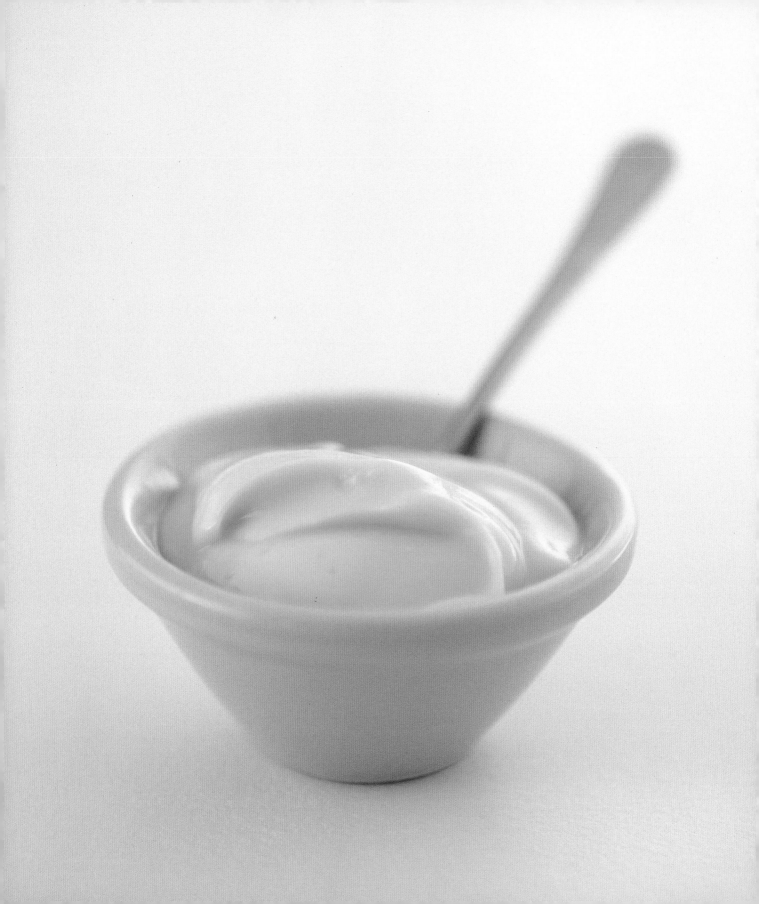

snacks

KATHY: I love Tamari Nuts and have a handful after breakfast and about 4 pm most days, detoxing or not. I might have a piece of fruit after lunch. That's it really. I don't normally eat between meals, so why do it when I am detoxing?

JAN: I tend to eat something for morning and afternoon tea because I find it helps prevent mid afternoon sugar cravings. I keep it pretty simple during the week – a small handful of our Tamari Nuts for morning tea and some fruit for afternoon tea, perhaps with a soy yoghurt depending on how energetic I've been during the day. On the weekend, I might enjoy a muesli ball or two, or one of our cookies with a cup of herbal tea or dandelion coffee.

One reason so many people struggle with excess weight is from indulging in the vast range of processed snack food on the market. Many of these products offer little in the way of nutritional value and offer mostly unnecessary fat and kilojoules. We like to keep the snacks simple and nutritious.

It makes good sense to have a healthy snack in between meals, especially if you hit an energy slump mid afternoon. We suggest you have a little snack mid morning, such as a tablespoon or two of Tamari Nuts (page 36) or perhaps a piece or two of fruit. This will help to sustain your energy through the morning and will have beneficial effects during the latter part of the day as well.

During a detox you do need to eat quite a few raw or lightly cooked vegetables. Our Spice, Nut & Seed Dip (page 34) is perfect for dipping vegetables into as a snack during the day. Or you can serve the dip along with our other savoury snacks for pre-dinner nibbles. You also don't have to miss out when it comes to sweet snacks because we've included several for you to enjoy any time of day, and they are all designed to help keep your energy at its best. Like any snacks, don't overdo them. These recipes are excellent to have on hand if you have friends drop by or if you need to take something to a friend's place.

spice, nut & seed dip with vegetables

This is a dukkah-like dipping mix to serve with carrot sticks, blanched asparagus or broccoli florets, green (spring) onions, red capsicum chunks or cherry tomatoes. Dip the vegetables in either extra virgin olive oil or stock before dipping in the spice mix for a light coating. You can also sprinkle this mix over soup, into salads or serve with bread.

55 g (1/3 cup) sesame seeds

3 tbsp coriander seeds

2 tbsp cumin seeds

55 g (1/3 cup) unsalted roasted cashews, finely chopped

1 tbsp dried thyme leaves

1/4 tsp salt

1/4 tsp freshly ground black pepper

1/4 tsp chilli powder

Toss sesame seeds in small saucepan over medium heat for 2 minutes or until lightly browned. Place in a bowl. Roast coriander and cumin seeds separately in pan over medium heat, tossing constantly for 30 seconds or until fragrant and just lightly browned. Place in a bowl to cool.

Use a spice or coffee grinder to grind coriander and cumin. Add to sesame seeds with cashews, thyme, salt, pepper and chilli. Mix well.

MAKES ABOUT 1 CUP

Spice mix will keep for up to 2 months in an airtight container.

spiced bran crackers

The Indian spices help create a wonderful more-ish flavour – it's difficult to leave them alone. They're excellent with Hummus (page 165), Green Olive & Lentil Dip (page 91) or Mushroom Paté (page 91) or Almond & Seed Spread (page 38) or to serve before dinner.

300 g (2 cups) all-purpose gluten-free
   flour mix

1 1/2 tsp ground coriander

1 tsp ground cumin

1/2 tsp chilli powder

1/2 tsp salt

1/2 tsp freshly ground black pepper

1/4 tsp gluten-free baking powder

25 g (1/4 cup) rice bran

2 tbsp extra virgin olive oil

Sift flour mix, coriander, cumin, chilli, salt, pepper and baking powder into a medium bowl. Stir in rice bran and make a well in the centre. Pour in 180 ml (3/4 cup) water and olive oil, and use a round-bladed knife in a cutting motion to mix ingredients together until clumps form. Use your hand to finish combining and bring mixture together into a firm dough. Knead in bowl until smooth.

Divide dough into 4 portions. Cover and set aside for 20 minutes to rest.

Roll a portion out between 2 sheets of baking paper until 2 mm thick. Use a 7 cm diameter round cutter to cut discs from the dough. Place on a large oven tray. Re-roll and cut dough scraps. Roll and cut remaining dough portions. Bake at 210°C for 11–12 minutes, swapping trays around halfway, or until lightly browned. Cool on trays.

MAKES ABOUT 28–30 CRACKERS

Crackers will keep for up to 3 weeks
if placed in layers in airtight container.

tamari nuts

Buy the freshest nuts you can from a shop that has a good turnover of stock. Use blanched or unblanched almonds. This is ideal to snack on during the day or to serve with a pre-dinner juice when entertaining.

120 g ($2/3$ cup) almond kernels

110 g ($2/3$ cup) raw cashews

100 g brazil nuts

55 g ($1/3$ cup) shelled pistachio nuts

COATING

2 tsp wheat-free tamari sauce

$1^{1}/2$ tsp honey

$1/2$ tsp sesame oil

$1/2$ tsp ground coriander

$1/4$ tsp chilli powder

Combine nuts and spread over an oven tray. Bake at 180°C, tossing halfway through cooking, for 14 minutes or until lightly browned.

Meanwhile, to make the Coating, combine all the ingredients in a medium heatproof bowl and mix well. Add the hot nuts straight from the oven and toss until the moisture evaporates and the nuts are lightly coated.

Spread the nuts on the tray and return to the oven for 1 minute. Cool on the tray (the coating will dry out and become a little crisp on cooling).

MAKES ABOUT 2$^{1}/2$ CUPS

Nuts will keep in an airtight container in a cool cupboard for up to 6 weeks.

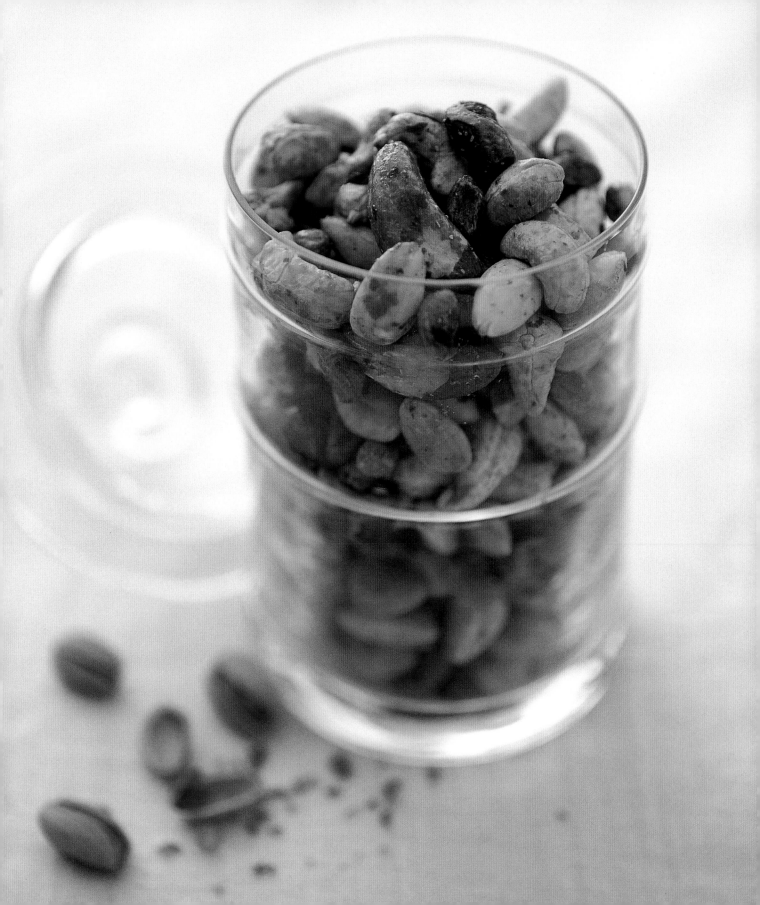

almond & seed spread

Excellent to have on crispbread or toast for breakfast or snacks. The nuts and seeds combined with crispbread or toast will provide a good protein source for vegetarians. And nuts and seeds are low GI (glycaemic index) – this means the spread will help provide you with sustained energy. Use your favourite nuts in different combinations for variety. Other nuts suitable include brazil nuts, pistachios, pecans, cashews, hazelnuts, pinenuts and macadamias.

400 g (2^1/2 cups) almond kernels

100 g (2/3 cup) pumpkin seed kernels

100 g (2/3 cup) sunflower seed kernels

55 g (1/3 cup) sesame seeds

light olive oil, canola oil or
  macadamia oil

sea salt (optional)

Spread almonds on an oven tray and roast at 180°C for 8 minutes, stirring after 4 minutes, or until almond kernels are lightly browned. Remove from oven. Spread pumpkin seed kernels, sunflower seeds and sesame seeds over another oven tray and roast for 5 minutes or until pumpkin seed kernels are lightly browned. Cool.

Process almonds and seeds in a food processor until finely ground. Add oil, a tablespoon at a time with the motor operating until a thick paste forms. Season with a pinch of sea salt, if using.

MAKES ABOUT 3 CUPS

Spread will keep for up to 2 months
in an airtight container in refrigerator.

salmon spread

A great topping for crispbread or our Gluten-free Flat Bread (page 23), this is a good snack for mid-afternoon when your energy might be lagging a little. You can also use canned pink salmon. Top with a few sunflower sprouts for added crunch.

1 x 210 g can red salmon, drained, skin
  and bones removed
1 lemon, rind finely grated, juiced
2 tbsp chopped fresh chives
1 tbsp chopped fresh flat-leaf parsley
1 tbsp finely diced red (Spanish) onion
2 tbsp Hummus (page 165)

Flake salmon in a small bowl with a fork. Add lemon rind, juice, chives, parsley, onion and Hummus and mix until well combined. Add a little extra lemon juice if needed, then season to taste.

MAKES ABOUT 250 ML (1 CUP)

Spread will keep for up to 2 days in
an airtight container in refrigerator.

cornmeal & berry muffins

Use your favourite berries in season in this recipe. If fresh berries aren't available, you can use frozen berries thawed on kitchen paper in refrigerator.

60 ml (1/4 cup) light olive oil or
   macadamia oil

3 eggs

1 x 140 g container apple fruit puree

125 ml (1/2 cup) soy milk or rice milk

2 1/2 tbsp honey

160 g fresh berries (such as
   raspberries, blueberries, mulberries,
   chopped strawberries, or a mixture of
   berries)

45 g (1/4 cup) polenta (yellow cornmeal)

250 g (1 2/3 cups) all-purpose gluten-
   free flour mix

3 1/2 tsp gluten-free baking powder

1 tsp ground cinnamon

Use a teaspoon or two of the oil to lightly grease 12 x 80 ml (1/3 cup) muffin pans. Line bases with baking paper if pans are not non-stick.

Whisk eggs, apple puree, soy or rice milk, honey and remaining oil in a large bowl until well combined. Stir in three-quarters of the berries with the polenta. Sift flour mix, baking powder and cinnamon over the top. Use a large metal spoon to fold through until well combined.

Spoon mixture into muffin pans and top with remaining berries. Bake at 180°C for 18 minutes or until lightly browned and a skewer inserted in the centres comes out clean. Stand in pan for 5 minutes before gently removing from pans and lifting onto a wire rack to cool. Serve warm or at room temperature.

MAKES 12

Muffins will keep in an airtight container for up to 2 days.
Warm before serving. Muffins can be frozen for up to 1 month.
Thaw in refrigerator and warm before serving.

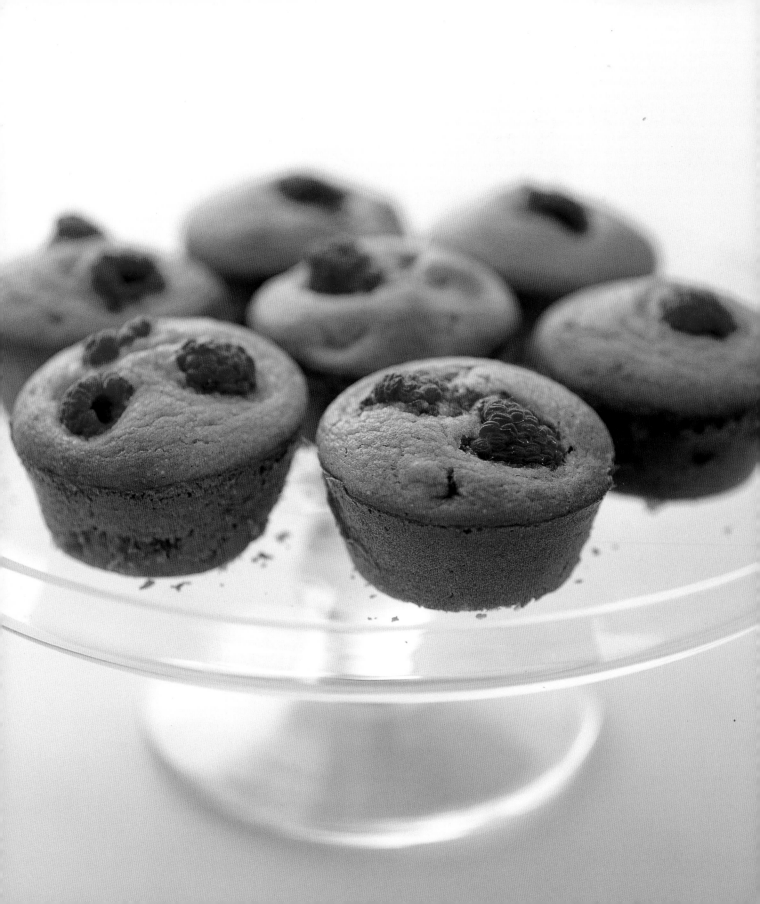

currant & nut ginger cookies

A bit like mini rock cakes because they are slightly cakey in texture, these are low in fat and sugar, and are very satisfying for an afternoon snack with a cup of herbal tea. You can use sultanas or chopped dried dates in place of currants if you prefer.

150 g (1 cup) all-purpose gluten-free
    flour mix

1 tsp gluten-free baking powder

1 tbsp ground ginger

90 g (1 cup) rolled oats

55 g (1/3 cup) dried currants

45 g (1/4 cup) chopped roasted unsalted
    cashews

40 g (1/4 cup) slivered almonds, toasted

60 ml (1/4 cup) rice syrup

2 tbsp light olive oil

2 eggs

Sift flour mix, baking powder and ginger into a large bowl. Stir in oats, currants, cashews and almonds. Whisk together rice syrup, oil, eggs and 2 tablespoons water until combined. Add to dry ingredients and mix well.

Drop heaped teaspoons of mixture onto 2 baking paper-lined oven trays. Use spoon to flatten mounds slightly. Bake at 200°C, swapping trays halfway through cooking, for 10 to 11 minutes or until golden brown. Cool on trays.

MAKES ABOUT 28

Cookies will keep for up to 1 week in an airtight container.

dried fruit, muesli & sesame balls

Choose muesli that contains little or no dried fruit (many dried fruits contain pres.... dates' label to ensure they are free of preservatives (generally they are preservative-free). This is a fabulous sweet treat to serve after dinner when entertaining or for that just-have-to-have-something-sweet craving in the mid-afternoon. The sweetness in the balls comes entirely from the dried fruit. You also benefit from the addition of muesli, which makes this an energy sustaining snack (excellent for those who have diabetes).

70 g ($^1/_2$ cup) chopped dried dates

60 g ($^1/_3$ cup) sultanas

$^1/_2$ tsp ground cinnamon

$^1/_4$ tsp ground nutmeg

$^1/_4$ tsp ground cardamom

205 g (2 cups) gluten-free muesli

30 g sesame seeds

Place dates, sultanas, 160 ml ($^2/_3$ cup) water and spices in a small saucepan and bring to the boil. Reduce heat to low, cover and simmer, stirring occasionally, for 9 minutes or until the fruit is soft and the remaining liquid is syrupy (don't overcook). Set aside to cool for 20 minutes.

Process muesli until finely chopped and place in a bowl. Place sesame seeds in saucepan and toss continually over high heat for 2–3 minutes or until light golden. Place on a plate.

Process cooked fruit mixture to a puree and add to muesli. Mix thoroughly with your hand to form a stiff mixture.

Roll 2 teaspoons of mixture into a ball (roughly the size of a cherry tomato) then toss in sesame seeds to coat. Repeat with remaining mixture and seeds.

MAKES ABOUT 22

Keep in an airtight container in refrigerator for up to 3 weeks.

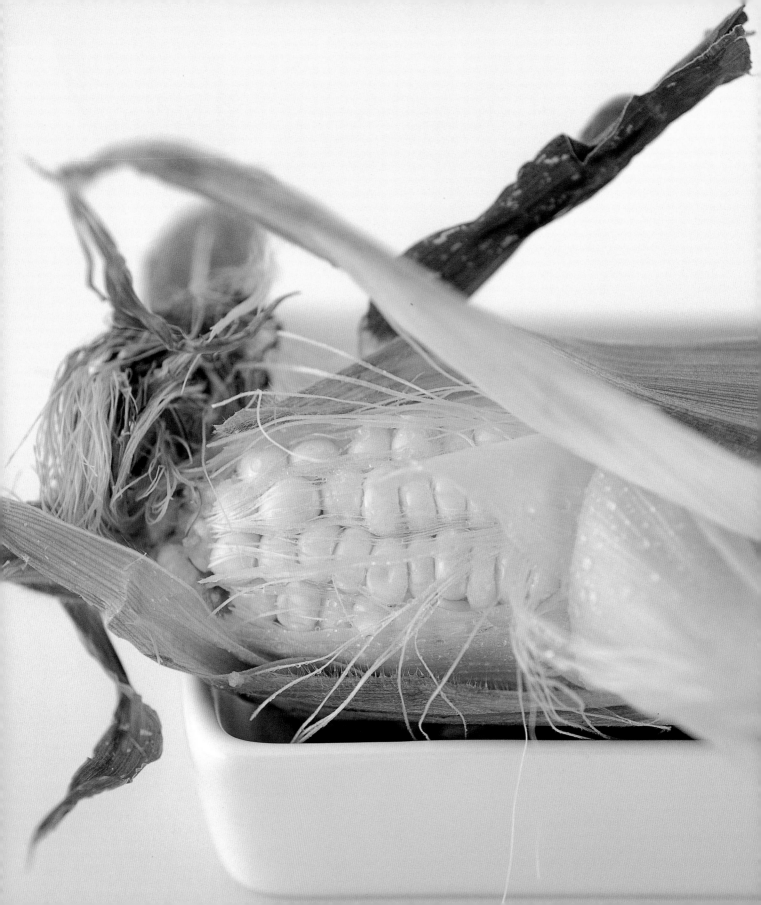

lunch

KATHY: Because I am not much of a breakfast girl, I get excited by the idea of lunch and start thinking about what I am going to eat at about 9 am. If I am working from home, then it's easy – usually some sort of big salad. On the weekends I will often make soup or cook lots of seafood to have with salad greens. If I am out for lunch and on the run, I usually look for an Asian-style takeaway and have a bowl of rice noodles with vegetables and chicken or tofu.

JAN: I usually make lunch to take to my clinic – a lunchbox filled with salad vegetables or roasted vegetables from the night before. If I don't have some cooked chicken, fish or lamb on hand, then I'll add some marinated tofu or canned salmon or tuna. I pack almonds or other nuts (a small container otherwise I'd keep eating them beyond a healthy amount!) and some fruit. I tend to snack between meals to keep good energy levels. If I buy lunch, it's usually fresh rice paper rolls or sushi rolls with miso or salad with some sort of protein.

These recipes are simple and easy to prepare and most can be made at the last minute. They rely on the use of the best and freshest ingredients and liberal servings of salad greens. Fresh herbs are a very important component of our recipes, partly for their nutritional value, but mostly for their flavour and you will find them in many of our recipes. Also, it's great to have a supply of stock in the freezer. The use of homemade stock will always improve the taste of a dish and you have the added advantage of knowing that it contains no additives. See Basics (page 158) for great stock recipes.

If you have to buy your lunch when detoxing, we suggest you look for a leafy tuna salad, rice with stir-fried vegetables and tofu, miso and sushi, rice noodles with chicken, lentil curry with rice, roast vegetables with fish or chicken, or ask for a container filled with salad ingredients from the sandwich bar (these won't have processed dressings on them) and a protein like salmon or chicken.

Many of the dishes in this chapter also double as an entree if you are entertaining. Just because you are detoxing doesn't mean you can't enjoy socialising with family and friends.

See page 93 for great recipes to take to work.

hot & sour chicken, noodle & tofu soup

You could use prawns instead of chicken. You will need about 600 g medium green prawns, peeled, deveined with tails left intact. This is an ideal lunch dish, or could be served as an entree before the Silver Bream en Papillote with Ginger & Eschallots (page 114).

2 L (8 cups) Chicken Stock (page 159)

1 stick fresh lemongrass, chopped

2 star anise

6 fresh kaffir lime leaves, bruised

3 cm piece ginger, sliced

2 small fresh red chillies, chopped

4 green (spring) onions, sliced on diagonal

2 vine-ripened tomatoes, each cut into 8 wedges

2 baby bok choy, trimmed, coarsely shredded

250 g skinless chicken breast fillet, thinly sliced crosswise

150 g firm tofu, cut into 2 cm pieces

¼ cup lime juice

100 g rice stick noodles, cooked according to directions on packet

2 tbsp fresh coriander leaves

2 tbsp fresh mint leaves

lime wedges, to serve

Combine stock, lemongrass, star anise, kaffir lime leaves and ginger in a large saucepan and simmer, uncovered, over medium heat until reduced by one third. Strain stock, discard solids and return stock to a clean pan. Add chillies, green onions, tomatoes and bok choy and simmer until bok choy is just wilted. Add sliced chicken, tofu and lime juice and simmer for 1–2 minutes until chicken is just cooked, then check seasoning. Place noodles in serving bowls, pour chicken soup over and sprinkle with herbs. Serve lime wedges on the side.

SERVES 4

Best made just before serving.

tuscan bean & vegetable soup with mint & olive salsa

The salsa adds a real boost of flavour to this soup, but it is also lovely without it. You can also use the salsa as a dip or as a topping for grilled fish or vegetables.

100 g (½ cup) dried cannellini beans, soaked in cold water overnight

1 tbsp olive oil

1 onion, sliced

2 L (8 cups) Chicken or Vegetable Stock (page 159)

4 cloves garlic, chopped

2 carrots, peeled and chopped

1 stick celery, chopped

6 egg (Roma) tomatoes, peeled, seeded and chopped

2 desiree potatoes, peeled and cut into 2 cm chunks

200 g green beans, trimmed and cut into 2 cm pieces

MINT & OLIVE SALSA

100 g Kalamata olives, pitted and chopped

4 green (spring) onions, chopped

½ cup fresh mint leaves, chopped

1 tbsp olive oil

1 tbsp lemon juice

To make Mint & Olive Salsa, combine all ingredients in a small food processor and process until just smooth, then season to taste.

Cook drained cannellini beans, uncovered, in simmering water about 30 minutes or until beans are tender. Drain.

Heat oil in a large saucepan and cook onion over low heat until soft, adding a little stock if onion is sticking to pan. Add stock, garlic, carrots, celery, tomatoes and potatoes, season to taste and simmer, uncovered, over medium heat about 35 minutes until vegetables are just tender. Add cooked cannellini beans, and green beans and simmer another 15 minutes.

Ladle soup into bowls and serve topped with a spoon of Mint & Olive Salsa.

SERVES 6–8

Salsa can be made 3 hours ahead.
Will keep, covered, in refrigerator.

pumpkin & garlic soup
with smoked tofu

You will find smoked tofu at health food stores, but if it's not available you can use spicy tofu or plain tofu. Grate it coarsely or shave it with a vegetable peeler.

4 slices gluten-free, rye or spelt bread, crusts removed

1 tbsp olive oil

1 onion, chopped

2 L (8 cups) Chicken or Vegetable Stock (page 159)

6 cloves garlic, chopped

1 kg pumpkin, peeled and chopped

80 g firm smoked tofu, shaved or coarsely grated

2 tbsp fresh coriander leaves

extra virgin olive oil, to drizzle

Cut bread into 1 cm pieces, place on an oven tray and bake at 200°C for 10 minutes or until crisp. Cool and store in an airtight container.

Heat oil in a large saucepan and cook onion over low heat until soft, adding a little stock if onion is sticking to pan. Add stock, garlic and pumpkin, then simmer, uncovered, about 40 minutes or until pumpkin is very soft. Remove from heat and puree mixture in a food processor, in batches, until smooth or use a hand blender to puree soup in pan. Season to taste and reheat.

Ladle soup into bowls and serve topped with croutons, tofu and coriander leaves, and drizzled with a little extra virgin olive oil.

SERVES 4

Soup and croutons can be made a day ahead. Soup will keep, covered, in refrigerator, croutons in an airtight container.

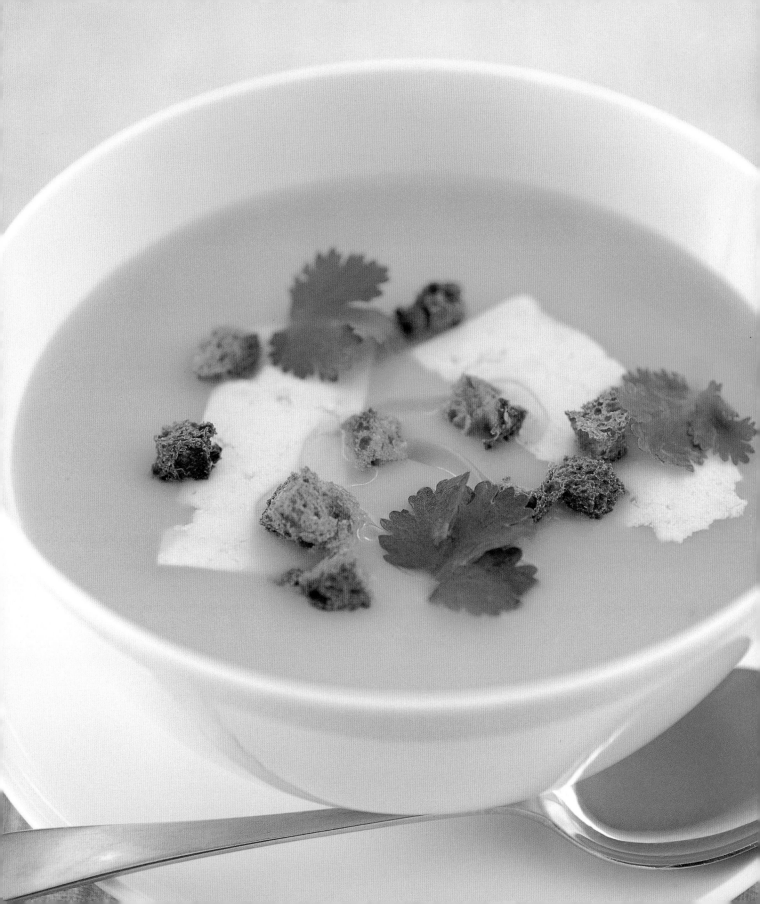

mediterranean prawn & mussel soup with herb polenta

If you are allergic to shellfish, then this soup is just as delicious made with a firm white fish such as blue eye or snapper instead of prawns and mussels. This Spanish-style soup uses almonds as a thickener, which also gives the soup a bit more body and at the same time adds wonderful texture and flavour.

olive oil

50 g blanched almonds

2 cloves garlic, peeled and flattened

1 small fresh red chilli

6 egg (Roma) tomatoes, peeled and seeded

1 Roasted Capsicum (page 163)

1 onion, chopped

2 L (8 cups) Fish or Chicken stock (pages 159 & 160)

pinch saffron, to taste

500 g mussels, scrubbed and bearded

500 g medium green prawns, peeled and deveined, tails intact

HERB POLENTA

150 g polenta (yellow cornmeal)

pinch cayenne, to taste

1/4 cup mixed chopped fresh herbs including basil, coriander, flat-leaf parsley

olive oil

To make Herb Polenta, bring 800 ml water to the boil, add salt to taste, reduce heat and add polenta in thin stream, then stir well. Reduce heat to very low, cover and cook about 20 minutes, stirring occasionally, until all the lumps are gone and polenta thickens and comes away from side of pan. Stir in cayenne and herbs, remove from heat, spoon onto a baking paper lined tray and shape into a 16 x 21 cm rectangle. When cold, cut into fingers and place on an oven tray. Set aside.

Heat 2 teaspoons olive oil in a frying pan and cook almonds, garlic and chilli over medium heat until almonds are golden. Combine almond mixture, half the tomatoes and half the capsicum in a food processor and process until smooth.

Heat 1 tablespoon oil in a large saucepan and cook onion over low heat until soft. Add tomato mixture, remaining finely chopped tomato and capsicum, stock and saffron and simmer, uncovered, over medium heat for 10 minutes. Add mussels, cover and simmer, about 5 minutes or until mussels have opened. Add prawns and simmer, uncovered, until prawns are just cooked, then season to taste.

Meanwhile brush polenta lightly with oil and grill on both sides until heated through. Ladle soup into bowls and serve with Herb Polenta.

SERVES 4

Polenta can be prepared a day ahead.
Will keep, covered, in refrigerator.

mushroom & chickpea soup with eggplant puree

This is a full bodied and earthy soup and we love the addition of a drizzle of truffle oil at the end — it feels quite decadent and makes it a special occasion dish.

1 small (about 275 g) eggplant

2 cloves garlic, chopped

2 tbsp plain soy yoghurt

1 tbsp lemon juice

100 g (½ cup) dried chickpeas, soaked in cold water overnight

2 bay leaves

1 tbsp olive oil

2 small leeks, trimmed, halved lengthwise and cut crosswise

1.5 L (6 cups) Chicken or Vegetable Stock (page 159)

500 g Swiss brown mushrooms, coarsely chopped

350 g silverbeet (stems discarded), shredded

truffle oil, to serve (optional)

Place eggplant on an oven tray and roast at 200°C for 30 minutes or until eggplant is very soft. Cool, then remove skin. Puree eggplant in a food processor with garlic, yoghurt and lemon juice until smooth, then season to taste.

Cook drained chickpeas, uncovered, in simmering water with bay leaves about 30 minutes or until tender. Drain and discard bay leaves.

Heat oil in a large saucepan and cook leeks over low heat until soft, adding a little stock if leeks are sticking to pan. Add stock, bring to the boil, then add mushrooms and simmer, uncovered, over medium heat for 10 minutes. Add chickpeas and simmer another 10 minutes, then stir in silverbeet, cook until just wilted and season to taste.

Ladle into soup bowls and serve topped with eggplant puree and a drizzle of truffle oil, if using.

SERVES 4–6

Eggplant puree can be made a day ahead.
Will keep, covered, in refrigerator.

asian-style duck salad

Duck breasts are very fatty and while that fat is delicious (according to Kathy), it's best removed when you are detoxing (so Jan says). You can toss calamari or roasted quail through this salad instead of duck and if you want to make it even more substantial, add some rice noodles.

2 large duck breasts (about 500 g),
  skin removed

1 carrot, peeled and cut into julienne

100 g snowpeas, trimmed and cut into
  julienne

100 g sugar snap peas, trimmed

1 large fresh red chilli, seeded and cut
  into julienne

200 g Chinese cabbage, finely shredded

100 g bean sprouts, trimmed

2 green (spring) onions, trimmed,
  halved and cut into julienne

1 cup firmly packed fresh coriander
  leaves

20 g (¼ cup) flaked almonds, toasted

extra coriander sprigs, to serve

DRESSING

1 tsp grated ginger

2 cloves garlic, finely chopped

60 ml (¼ cup) lime juice

1 tsp sesame oil

1 tbsp wheat-free tamari sauce

¼ tsp honey

To make dressing, combine all ingredients and check seasoning.

Heat a non-stick frying pan and cook duck breasts over medium heat about 3 minutes each side, depending on thickness, until golden (this will give you pink duck). Remove from pan, cover loosely with foil and stand for 10 minutes before thinly slicing crosswise.

Combine carrot, snowpeas, sugar snap peas and chilli in a bowl and pour boiling water over. Drain immediately and rinse under cold water. Return to bowl, add cabbage, bean sprouts, green onion, coriander, almonds and duck, and toss to combine. Toss half the dressing with salad and place in shallow bowls. Top with extra coriander sprigs, then drizzle with remaining dressing.

SERVES 4 FOR LUNCH OR 6 AS AN ENTREE

Dressing can be made 3 hours ahead and kept, covered, at room temperature. Salad best made just before serving.

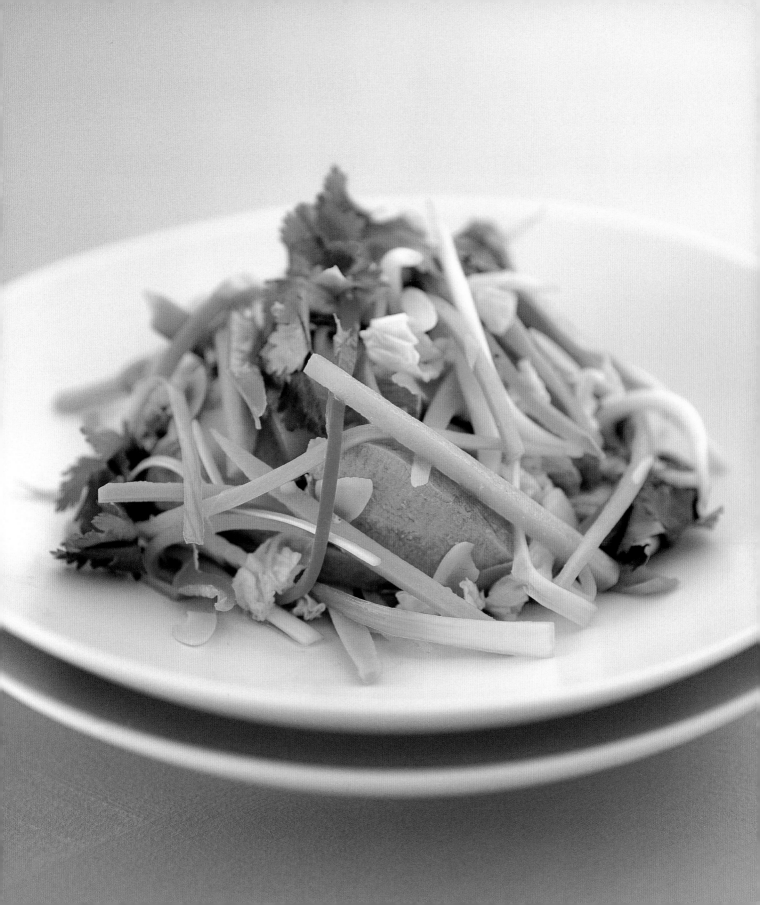

roasted quail with quinoa salad & grilled figs

If you haven't tried quinoa before you are in for a treat. It's a high-protein ancient grain that is excellent served both hot or cold. It has a chewy texture and a lovely nutty flavour, but benefits from the addition of herbs or being cooked in stock. You will find it in health food stores. If fresh figs are not available, use sliced ripe pears. This dish is pictured on the cover.

4 large quails

extra virgin olive oil

190 g (1 cup) quinoa

500 ml (2 cups) Chicken Stock
(page 159)

6 green (spring) onions, chopped

1 cup firmly packed fresh flat-leaf
parsley

2 tbsp pinenuts, toasted

2 tbsp currants

1 tsp grated lemon rind

1 tbsp lemon juice

4 figs, halved

Brush quails with a little oil and cook over high heat in a non-stick frying pan until golden all over, then place on an oven tray. Roast at 200°C for 10 minutes until tender. Rest in a warm place for 10 minutes, then cut each quail into 4 pieces.

Meanwhile, combine quinoa and chicken stock in a saucepan, add salt to taste and bring to the boil, then simmer, covered, over medium heat about 15 minutes or until most of the stock is absorbed and quinoa is tender. Remove lid and stir over heat until all stock is evaporated. Remove from heat and cool.

Add green onions, parsley, pinenuts, currants, lemon rind and juice and 1 tablespoon oil to cooled quinoa, season to taste and stir to combine.

Brush figs lightly with oil and chargrill or grill until golden.

Serve quartered quail on a bed of quinoa salad with chargrilled figs to one side.

SERVES 4

Best made just before serving.

blackened chicken with coleslaw & guacamole

If you can't find a Cajun spice mix in your local supermarket, it's easy enough to make one yourself. Try a mixture of sweet paprika, salt, dried thyme, cayenne pepper and a little dried onion and garlic – that way you can make it as mild or as hot as you like. You can also rub this mixture onto salmon or snapper fillets before you pan fry them.

4 skinless chicken thigh fillets,
  trimmed of any fat

olive oil

2 tbsp Cajun spice mix, or to taste

300 g red cabbage, thinly shredded

300 g Chinese cabbage, thinly shredded

6 green (spring) onions, sliced
  diagonally

1/2 cup fresh coriander leaves

1/4 cup Light Mayonnaise (page 164)

lemon wedges, to serve

GUACAMOLE

1 avocado, cut into 1 cm pieces

2 tbsp lemon juice

1/2 large fresh red chilli, seeded, finely
  chopped

For Guacamole, combine ingredients, mash coarsely with a fork and season to taste.

Brush chicken lightly with oil and toss in Cajun spice mix.

Combine red and Chinese cabbage in a bowl, toss with 1/2 teaspoon salt and stand for 30 minutes. Toss cabbage mixture, green onions, coriander and Light Mayonnaise, and check seasoning.

Heat a non-stick frying pan and cook chicken over medium heat on both sides until cooked through. Serve chicken on a bed of coleslaw with Guacamole and lemon wedges to one side.

SERVES 4

Guacamole can be made 1 hour ahead.
Will keep, covered, in refrigerator.

chicken kebabs with baby spinach & pomegranate salad

Pomegranate seeds look like little pink jewels and are a wonderful addition to a salad. They are in season around April and May and there really is no substitute, although you could add some chopped mango if you were making this dish in summer.

4 skinless chicken thigh fillets,
    trimmed of any fat and cut into 3 cm
    pieces

extra virgin olive oil

pomegranate molasses

4 bamboo skewers, soaked in cold
    water 30 minutes

100 g snowpeas, trimmed and halved
    lengthwise

2 zucchini, thinly sliced lengthwise and
    halved crosswise

150 g baby spinach leaves

1 avocado, seeded, peeled and cut into
    2 cm pieces

1 pomegranate, halved and seeds
    removed

1 tbsp pumpkin seed kernels, toasted

1 tbsp pinenuts, toasted

Toss chicken pieces with 1 tablespoon each of olive oil and pomegranate molasses, season to taste, then thread onto bamboo skewers.

Combine snowpeas and zucchini in a bowl, pour boiling water over, then drain and rinse under cold water. Pat dry with absorbent paper.

Combine 1 tablespoon oil and 1 teaspoon pomegranate molasses and season to taste. Combine snowpeas, zucchini, spinach leaves, avocado and pomegranate seeds and toss gently with dressing.

Chargrill or grill chicken kebabs over medium heat on both sides until cooked. Serve salad topped with chicken kebabs and sprinkled with pumpkin seed kernels and pinenuts.

SERVES 4

Best made just before serving

chicken, broad bean & mango salad

This is a fresh, light and easy-to-prepare salad that makes use of leftover poached chicken. You can also substitute cooked prawns or seared calamari for the chicken. Late October, early November you will find both broad beans and mango in season, however when summer arrives and the broad beans disappear, you might like to substitute baby beans.

12 chat potatoes

500 g broad beans, podded

1 small avocado, seeded, peeled and
   cut into 2 cm pieces

1 small mango, peeled and cut into
   2 cm pieces

1/2 Poached Chicken (page 161)

1 bunch rocket, trimmed

2 tbsp dill or coriander sprigs

1 tbsp extra virgin olive oil

1 tbsp lemon juice

Cook potatoes, uncovered, in simmering salted water until tender. Drain, cool and halve lengthwise. Cook broad beans in simmering salted water, uncovered, for 3 minutes. Drain, rinse under cold water, then peel.

Combine potatoes and broad beans and divide among plates, then top with avocado and mango. Remove skin from chicken, tear chicken into bite-sized pieces and place in centre of salad. Toss rocket, dill or coriander, oil and lemon juice, season to taste and serve on top of chicken.

SERVES 4

Best made just before serving.

stir-fried lamb with asian greens & rice noodles

Don't slice the lamb too thinly as you want it to retain its shape when you cook it. You could use other types of Asian-style greens if you like, such as choy sum or gai lan.

600 g lamb backstraps (eye of loin),
　　sliced into 1 cm thick slices

soy sauce or wheat-free tamari sauce

1 tsp sesame oil

light olive oil

3 eschallots, cut into wedges

2 cloves garlic, chopped

2 tsp grated ginger

125 ml ($1/2$ cup) Chicken Stock (page 159)

1 bunch Chinese broccoli, trimmed and
　　sliced crosswise into 4

1 bunch broccolini, trimmed and halved
　　crosswise

1 large fresh red chilli, sliced

2 tbsp lime juice

125 g rice vermicelli noodles, cooked

4 green (spring) onions, sliced on the
　　diagonal

$1/3$ cup fresh coriander sprigs

35 g ($1/4$ cup) cashews, toasted and
　　coarsely chopped

Rub lamb with 1 teaspoon soy sauce and sesame oil. Heat 1 tablespoon oil in a non-stick wok and stir-fry lamb over high heat in batches until just cooked, then remove from wok.

Add a little more oil to wok if necessary, then add eschallots, garlic and ginger and stir-fry for 1 minute, then add stock. Add broccoli stems and broccolini, stir-fry for 30 seconds, then cover and cook over low heat for 1 minute. Add broccoli leaves and stir-fry until wilted. Add chilli, lime juice and 1 tablespoon soy sauce and stir-fry another minute.

Cook noodles according to directions on packet and place in serving bowls. Top with vegetable mixture, lamb and any lamb juices, then sprinkle with sliced green onions, coriander and cashews.

SERVES 4

Best made just before serving.

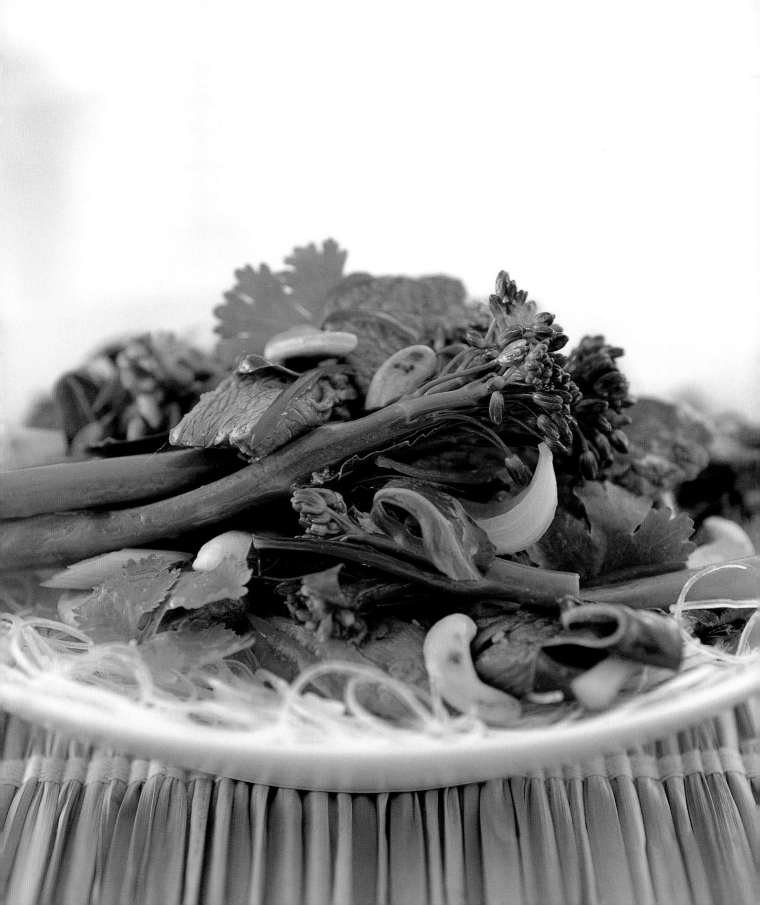

marinated lamb with corn, zucchini & polenta fritters

If you want to eat lamb when you are detoxing, then we suggest that you only eat organic lamb that has been trimmed of all fat and have it just once a week. These gorgeous fritters are ideal served as a breakfast or brunch dish with grilled mushrooms and roasted tomatoes, or serve them with smoked salmon and a handful of baby salad leaves.

600 g lamb backstraps (eye of loin), cut
  into 3 cm pieces

2 tsp sumac

4 bamboo skewers, soaked in cold water
  for 30 minutes

olive oil

1 bunch rocket, trimmed

1 avocado, seeded, peeled and chopped

lemon wedges, to serve

TOMATO SALSA

3 vine-ripened tomatoes, seeded, finely
  chopped

1/2 small red (Spanish) onion, finely
  chopped

2 tbsp shredded fresh basil

CORN, ZUCCHINI & POLENTA FRITTERS

1 corn cob

1 zucchini

85 g (1/2 cup) polenta (yellow cornmeal)

35 g (1/4 cup) chickpea flour (besan)

1/2 tsp bicarbonate of soda

1/2 cup soy milk

2 tsp butter, melted

1 egg, separated

For Tomato Salsa, combine all ingredients and season to taste.

Toss lamb with sumac, cover and stand at room temperature for 30 minutes.

To make Corn, Zucchini & Polenta Fritters, using a small serrated knife, remove kernels from corn cob. Coarsely grate zucchini. Combine polenta, chickpea flour and bicarbonate of soda in a bowl and stir in soy milk, butter and egg yolk. Add corn and zucchini, season to taste, then fold in lightly whisked egg white.

Lightly grease a non-stick frying pan and cook scant 1/4 cupfuls of batter over medium heat about 2 minutes or until browned underneath. Turn and cook other side. Repeat with remaining batter. Place fritters on a plate and cover with a clean tea towel while cooking all the batter.

Meanwhile, thread lamb onto skewers, brush with a little oil and pan fry, turning occasionally until cooked.

Serve fritters with lamb skewers, tomato salsa, rocket, avocado and lemon wedges.

SERVES 4
MAKES 8 FRITTERS

Tomato Salsa can be made 1 hour ahead.
Will keep, covered, at room temperature.

lamb backstrap with chickpea & eggplant salad

We like to serve our lamb pink, so you will need to increase the cooking times a little if you prefer well done. Resting all meats, chicken and fish is very important before serving. This allows the juices to set and you will have a more tender and juicy result. It also makes it easier to carve.

100 g (½ cup) dried chickpeas, soaked in cold water overnight

1 eggplant, cut into 2 cm pieces

2 red (Spanish) onions, each cut into 8 wedges

4 egg (Roma) tomatoes, halved lengthwise, then crosswise

2 zucchini, cut crosswise into 2 cm thick slices

extra virgin olive oil

2 tbsp fresh thyme leaves

1 tbsp red wine vinegar or balsamic vinegar

600 g lamb backstraps

125 ml (½ cup) Yoghurt Dressing (page 164), to serve

fresh thyme sprigs, to serve

Baby Spinach Salad (page 162), to serve

Cook drained chickpeas in simmering water about 30 minutes or until tender. Drain and rinse under cold water.

Place eggplant, onions, tomatoes and zucchini on an oven tray and toss with a little oil. Season to taste and roast at 200°C for 30 minutes, turning once, or until browned and tender. Remove from oven and cool slightly.

Combine vegetables, chickpeas and half the thyme with 1 tablespoon oil and vinegar, season to taste and toss gently.

Brush lamb with a little olive oil and rub with remaining thyme leaves. Pan fry lamb in a hot non-stick frying pan until golden, then place on an oven tray and roast at 200°C about 10 minutes for pink lamb. Rest in a warm place for 10 minutes, before slicing on the diagonal.

Top Chickpea & Eggplant Salad with sliced lamb. Drizzle with Yoghurt Dressing and sprinkle with sprigs of thyme. Serve with Baby Spinach Salad.

SERVES 4

Chickpea & Eggplant Salad can be made a day ahead.
Will keep, covered, in refrigerator.

peppered venison with beetroot salsa & asparagus

We love venison and it is just so good for you. It's very low in fat, so serve it rare or medium rare – it's best not to overcook it. The venison farmed in Australia tends to have a mild flavour and is not as gamey as you would find in New Zealand or Europe.

4 x 100 g venison leg steaks

extra virgin olive oil

1 tsp cracked black pepper

12 spears asparagus, trimmed

130 g snowpeas, trimmed and halved
   lengthwise

1 bunch rocket, trimmed

1 tbsp lemon juice

1/2 cup Tahini Dressing (page 164),
   to serve

BEETROOT SALSA

2 large beetroot, trimmed and halved

1 tbsp olive oil

1 tbsp balsamic vinegar

2 tbsp chopped fresh mint or chives

For Beetroot Salsa, wrap beetroot in foil, place on an oven tray and roast at 200°C for 50–60 minutes until beetroot are tender. Remove foil and, when cool enough to handle, peel away skin. Cut beetroot into 1 cm cubes, combine with remaining ingredients and season to taste.

Brush venison steaks with a little oil and sprinkle with cracked black pepper. Chargrill steaks over medium to high heat for 2–3 minutes each side or until cooked to your liking, then rest, loosely covered, in a warm place for 10 minutes. Slice each steak across the grain, into three pieces.

Blanch asparagus and snowpeas in simmering salted water for 2 minutes. Drain, rinse under cold water and pat dry with absorbent paper.

Toss rocket with 1 tablespoon oil and lemon juice and season to taste. Top rocket with asparagus, snowpeas and venison and spoon Beetroot Salsa around plate. Serve with Tahini Dressing.

SERVES 4

Beetroot Salsa can be made a day ahead.
Will keep, covered, in refrigerator.

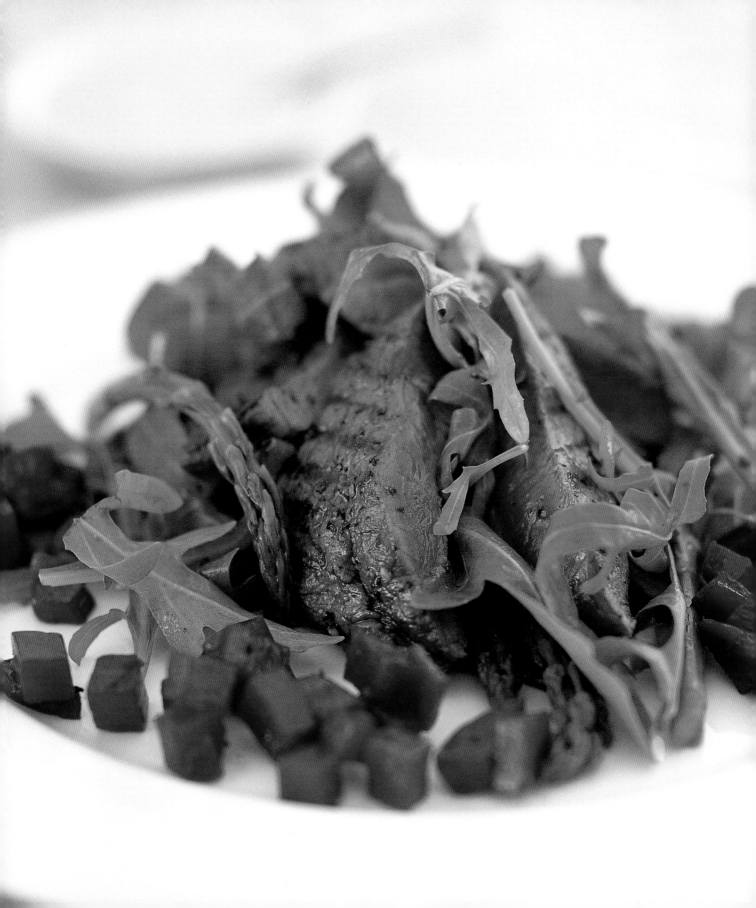

fennel, leek & scallop risotto

The best risotto is always made with homemade stock and stirred continuously. Some food writers cook it by the absorption method but it's just not the same.

olive oil

1 small leek, white part only, chopped

400 g fennel bulb, trimmed, cored and
  finely chopped

1 L (4 cups) Fish or Chicken Stock
  (pages 159 & 160), approximately

1 clove garlic, chopped

300 g (1 1/2 cups) arborio rice

2 tsp butter

1 tbsp chopped fresh dill

20 large scallops, without roe

Heat 1 tablespoon oil in a large saucepan and cook leek and fennel, covered, over low heat until soft, adding a little stock if vegetables are sticking to pan. Add garlic and rice and stir over medium heat until rice is coated and toasted lightly. Have stock simmering in another saucepan.

Add 250 ml (1 cup) stock and stir over heat until stock is absorbed. Add remaining stock 125 ml (1/2 cup) at a time, stirring constantly, allowing each addition to be absorbed before adding the next. With last addition of stock, add butter and two thirds of the dill and season to taste. Remove from heat, cover and stand 5 minutes.

Brush scallops with a little oil and chargrill on both sides until just cooked. Transfer to a plate.

Spoon risotto into shallow bowls and serve topped with scallops and their juices and remaining dill.

SERVES 4 AS A MAIN COURSE or 6 AS AN ENTREE

Best made just before serving.

seafood antipasto

If you are having it for lunch, serve it with a Leafy Green Salad (page 161). Place each little pile of seafood around the plate and put a few leaves in the middle. It's a wonderful mix of delicate flavours.

extra virgin olive oil

lemon wedges and baby salad leaves or
  watercress sprigs, to serve

CHARGRILLED SCALLOPS WITH HUMMUS

8 large scallops, without roe

1/3 cup Hummus (page 165)

1 tsp fresh thyme leaves

STEAMED PRAWNS WITH LEEK PUREE

1 leek, trimmed and sliced into 1 cm rings

60 ml (1/2 cup) Chicken Stock (page 159)
  or water

8 large cooked prawns, peeled and deveined,
  tails intact

1 tsp fresh dill sprigs

SQUID WITH CHERRY TOMATOES

4 baby squid, cleaned

1 large fresh red chilli, sliced

1 clove garlic, chopped

16 cherry tomatoes, halved

SMOKED SALMON, AVOCADO
& JULIENNE CUCUMBER

1/2 avocado, seeded, peeled and finely chopped

1 Lebanese (small green) cucumber, peeled,
  halved lengthways, seeded
  and cut into julienne

1 tbsp lemon juice

200 g sliced smoked salmon

To make Chargrilled Scallops with Hummus, brush scallops with a little oil and chargrill over high heat about 30 seconds each side or until just cooked. Spoon Hummus onto plates and top with a scallop and thyme leaves. Season to taste.

To make Steamed Prawns with Leek Puree, combine leek, 2 teaspoons oil and stock or water in a saucepan, cover and cook over low heat until leek is soft. Remove lid and cook until all liquid is evaporated. Season to taste and puree with a hand-held blender until smooth. Place prawns in the top of a steamer over a pan of simmering water, cover and steam about 1 minute until prawns are just cooked. Spoon leek puree onto plates and top with prawns and a few sprigs of dill.

To make Squid with Cherry Tomatoes, halve squid lengthwise and score inside surface. Heat 1 tablespoon oil in a frying pan and cook squid about 1 minute over high heat or until curled and just cooked. Remove from pan, add chilli, garlic and tomatoes and cook over high heat for 1 minute. Return squid to pan, toss to combine, season to taste and spoon onto plates.

To make Smoked Salmon, Avocado & Julienne Cucumber, place avocado onto plates, top with cucumber and drizzle with lemon juice. Lay smoked salmon over the top.

Serve with a few baby salad leaves or sprigs of watercress and lemon wedges.

SERVES 4

Leek puree can be made a day ahead.
Will keep, covered, in refrigerator.

prawn, fennel &
pink grapefruit salad

This salad is gorgeous for a light lunch in autumn or winter just as it is, or you could cook a mixture of prawns and calamari. In that case, use half the number of prawns and add 2 cleaned calamari, cut into rings. If baby fennel is not available, use a regular fennel bulb, but you might not need all of it. A mandolin, or V-slicer as they are sometimes called, is the best gadget to use for shaving the fennel, but if you don't have one you can use a vegetable peeler or just cut it very thinly with a sharp knife. You can add chunks of avocado to the salad if you like.

1 tbsp olive oil

24 medium green prawns, peeled and
   deveined, tails intact

1 tbsp white wine vinegar or lemon
   juice

100 g rocket leaves

2 pink grapefruit, peeled and
   segmented

2 baby fennel, trimmed and shaved with
   a mandolin

1 tbsp fresh dill sprigs

2 tsp salt-packed capers, rinsed

Heat oil in a heavy-based non-stick frying pan and stir-fry prawns, in batches, over medium heat until just cooked, adding a little more oil if necessary. Remove from pan and place in a bowl.

Remove pan from heat, deglaze pan with vinegar or lemon juice, season to taste, then pour mixture over prawns.

Place rocket leaves on a large platter, top with grapefruit, fennel and prawns and their dressing. Sprinkle with dill and capers.

SERVES 8 AS AN ENTREE or 4 AS A LIGHT MEAL

Best made just before serving.

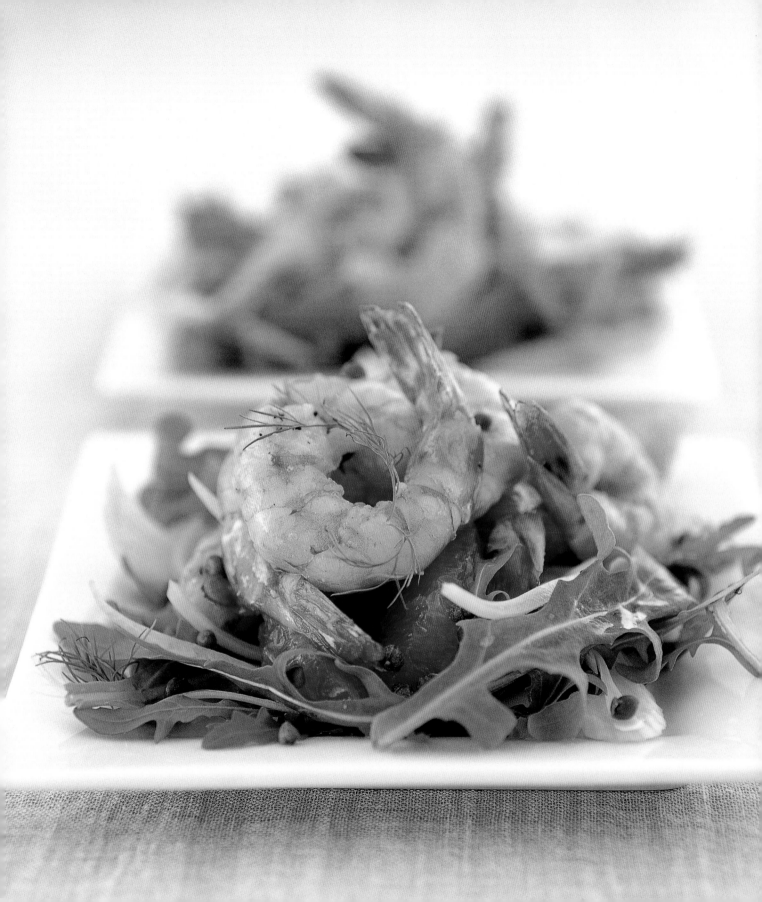

spicy blue eye &
green pawpaw stir-fry

Any firm white fish is suitable for this recipe. You could also use green mango instead of pawpaw. We like to marinate the fish in its coating for an hour to develop the flavours, but if you don't have the time, just coat it and cook it – it's still delicious.

1/2 tsp belacan (dried shrimp paste)

1/4 tsp ground turmeric

2 cloves garlic, crushed

1 tsp grated ginger

2 tsp rice-wine vinegar

600 g blue eye, cut into 2 cm pieces

light olive oil

50 g (1 cup) bean sprouts

150 g green pawpaw, seeded, peeled
   and cut into julienne

6 green (spring) onions, cut into 2 cm
   lengths, halved lengthwise

1/2 cup fresh coriander sprigs

1/2 cup fresh dill sprigs

1/2 cup fresh Thai basil leaves

4 butter lettuce leaves, to serve

Chilli Sauce (page 166) and lime
   wedges, to serve

Crumble belacan into a dry non-stick pan and stir over medium heat about 2 minutes until fragrant. Combine belacan, turmeric, garlic, ginger and rice-wine vinegar in a bowl, add blue eye and toss to coat, then cover and refrigerate for 1 hour. Bring to room temperature.

Heat 1 tablespoon oil in a non-stick wok and stir-fry fish over medium heat until just cooked, then remove from pan. Add a little more oil to pan if necessary and stir-fry bean sprouts and pawpaw over high heat for 30 seconds. Add green onions and herbs and stir-fry another 10 seconds or until herbs are just wilted.

Place pawpaw and bean sprout mixture in lettuce cups and serve topped with fish. Serve with chilli sauce and lime wedges.

SERVES 4

Best made just before serving.

smoked trout salad with apple, walnuts & witlof

Salmon roe, or salmon pearls as they are sometimes called, were once an exotic ingredient. Now they are available from fish markets and food halls and add a fabulous burst of the flavour of the sea to any dish in which they are used. If you can't get salmon roe, top this salad with a little julienne of smoked salmon, or just leave it out. If you'd like a slightly lower fat version of this recipe, use Yoghurt Dressing (page 164) in place of Light Mayonnaise.

2 x 300 g smoked trout

1 green apple, peeled, cored and cut into 2 cm pieces

1 stick celery, finely chopped

$^{1}/_{2}$ avocado, seeded, peeled and cut into 2 cm pieces

1 Lebanese (small green) cucumber, peeled, halved lengthwise, seeded and cut into 2 cm pieces

4 radishes, thinly sliced

35 g ($^{1}/_{3}$ cup) walnuts, roasted and coarsely chopped

60 ml ($^{1}/_{4}$ cup) Light Mayonnaise (page 164)

2 witlof, leaves separated

1 cup watercress leaves

1 tbsp extra virgin olive oil

1 tbsp verjuice or lemon juice

2 tbsp salmon roe

1 tbsp fresh chervil leaves

Remove skin and bones from trout and break into 2 cm pieces. Combine trout, apple, celery, avocado, cucumber, radishes, walnuts and mayonnaise and toss gently.

Toss witlof and watercress with olive oil and verjuice or lemon juice and top with smoked trout mixture. Serve salad sprinkled with salmon roe and chervil.

SERVES 4

Best made just before serving.

salmon & broad bean salad with preserved lemon dressing

Preserved lemons are available from delicatessens and food stores, but it's very easy to do yourself, especially in winter when lemons are at their best, plentiful and cheap. Pack quartered lemons into a sterilised jar with salt to cover, a bay leaf and a cinnamon stick, cover tightly and leave for at least a month before using.

400 g salmon fillets, skinned and
  pinboned
300 g kipfler or other waxy potatoes,
  scrubbed
500 g broad beans, podded
200 g baby beans, topped
1/4 preserved lemon, rinsed
2 tbsp chopped fresh chives
1 tbsp extra virgin olive oil
1 tbsp lemon juice
40 g (1/4 cup) caperberries
2 cups watercress sprigs

Line a steaming basket with baking paper and top with salmon. Place basket over a pan of simmering water, cover and steam for 3–5 minutes depending on thickness, until salmon is just cooked and still a little pink in the centre. Rest for 30 minutes before breaking into large chunks.

Cook potatoes, uncovered, in simmering salted water until tender. Drain and, when cool enough to handle, peel and slice.

Cook broad beans and baby beans, uncovered, in simmering salted water for 3 minutes, drain and rinse under cold water. Slip skins off broad beans.

Remove and discard flesh from preserved lemon. Chop skin finely. Combine preserved lemon, chives, oil and lemon juice and season to taste.

Place sliced potatoes on plates, top with caperberries, watercress and baby beans, then chunks of salmon. Spoon broad beans around plate and drizzle with dressing.

SERVES 4

Best made just before serving.

steamed mussels with caper & chilli gremolata

When choosing mussels, always buy the black ones. Soak mussels in cold water for 1 hour before giving them a good scrub and pulling off their beards. Throw away any that are damaged or that are open and will not close when tapped. You only want to cook live mussels.

1 tbsp olive oil

1 eschallot, finely chopped

1 kg black mussels, scrubbed and
   bearded

60 ml (¼ cup) Chicken Stock
   (page 159) or water

Leafy Green Salad (page 161) and
   gluten-free, spelt or rye bread, to
   serve

CAPER & CHILLI GREMOLATA

1 tbsp drained capers, chopped

1 large fresh red chilli, seeded and
   chopped

2 cloves garlic, finely chopped

2 tbsp chopped fresh flat-leaf parsley

To make Caper & Chilli Gremolata, combine all ingredients and season to taste.

Heat oil in a large saucepan and cook eschallot over low heat until soft. Add mussels and stock or water and cook, covered, over medium heat about 5 minutes or until all mussels have opened. Discard any mussels that do not open.

Serve mussels and their broth in deep bowls and sprinkle with Caper and Chilli Gremolata.

Serve with Leafy Green Salad and bread.

SERVES 4

Best made just before serving.

butterflied sardines in vine leaves with eggplant

Sardines are high in omega 3 fatty acids, which are wonderful anti-inflammatory agents in the body. Not only are omega 3s good for reducing inflammation, they also help reduce your risk of cardiovascular disease. As a bonus, you can eat the bones in sardines, making them a good source of calcium. Ask your fishmonger to butterfly the sardines for you.

450 g eggplant, cut into 8 slices

olive oil

1 x 400 g can tomatoes

2 cloves garlic, chopped

1/2 cup chopped mixed fresh herbs
  including mint, flat-leaf parsley, basil
  and coriander

1 tbsp pinenuts, roasted and chopped

16 butterflied sardines

8 vine leaves in brine, rinsed

Leafy Green Salad (page 161) and
  lemon wedges, to serve

Place eggplant on an oven tray, brush with a little oil and grill on both sides until golden.

Combine chopped tomatoes and their juice and garlic in a saucepan and cook, uncovered, over medium heat until thick, then season to taste.

Combine herbs and pinenuts. Lay half the sardines, skin side down on work surface and top with herb mixture. Lay the other sardines over, skin side up. Trim vine leaves if too large. Wrap a vine leaf around each sardine parcel, leaving open at both ends, and secure with a toothpick. Brush vine leaves with a little oil and grill, barbecue or chargrill about 1 minute each side or until just brown.

Place eggplant on serving plates. Spoon tomato mixture over eggplant, top with sardines in vine leaves and serve with Leafy Green Salad and lemon wedges.

SERVES 4 FOR LUNCH or 8 AS AN ENTREE

Tomato sauce can be made a day ahead. Will keep, covered, in refrigerator.

steamed cuttlefish with caramelised onions & puy lentils

Ask your fishmonger to clean the cuttlefish, but make sure you see it first. You want to be certain it is very fresh. As with all our recipes, the freshness and quality of the produce is the key to the dish's flavour, especially with such a simple form of cooking as steaming.

4 (1 kg) cuttlefish, cleaned

2 tsp grated lemon rind

2 tbsp lemon juice

1 tbsp extra virgin olive oil

200 g (1 cup) French green (Puy) lentils

1 cup firmly packed fresh mixed herbs, including coriander, mint, basil and flat-leaf parsley

CARAMELISED ONIONS

1 tbsp olive oil

2 red (Spanish) onions, thinly sliced

60 ml (¼ cup) Chicken Stock (page 159) or water

1 tbsp balsamic vinegar

½ tsp honey

To make Caramelised Onions, heat oil in a saucepan, add onion and stock or water and cook, covered, over low heat about 20 minutes or until onions are very soft. Add vinegar and honey and cook, uncovered, stirring occasionally, until onions are caramelised, then season to taste.

Using a thin-bladed fish knife, shave cuttlefish lengthwise into 2mm thick slices. Place cuttlefish in the top of a double steamer and steam over simmering water about 30 seconds or until just cooked. Transfer to a bowl and stir in lemon rind, juice and oil.

Cook lentils in simmering water about 15–20 minutes or until tender. Drain and rinse under cold water, then return to pan and stir in caramelised onions. Check seasoning.

Toss cuttlefish mixture with herbs and serve on a bed of lentil mixture.

SERVES 4

Caramelised onion and lentil mixture can be made 3 hours ahead. Will keep, covered, at room temperature.

seared tuna & asparagus salad with tamari dressing

Don't attempt to make this salad unless you use the best quality sashimi tuna and make sure you only sear the surface – you are not trying to cook it through. You can substitute seared prawns or chargrilled quail for the tuna. Both taste just as delicious with this salad.

1 large fresh red chilli, seeded and cut
　into julienne

2 green (spring) onions, trimmed and
　cut into julienne

600 g piece of sashimi-quality tuna

olive oil

sea salt

cracked black pepper

12 spears asparagus, trimmed

150 g sugar snap peas, trimmed

150 g baby salad leaves

1 Roasted Capsicum (page 163)

1/4 cup fresh basil

1/4 cup fresh coriander leaves

2 tbsp flaked almonds, toasted

TAMARI DRESSING

1 tbsp olive oil

1 tbsp lime juice

1 tbsp wheat-free tamari sauce

1 clove garlic, finely chopped

To make Tamari Dressing, combine all ingredients and season to taste. Stand for 30 minutes for flavours to develop.

Cover chilli and green onion with chilled water for 30 minutes, then drain.

Brush tuna with oil, then rub with sea salt and plenty of cracked black pepper. Heat a heavy-based frying pan until very hot and sear tuna on all sides about 20 seconds or until only the surface of the tuna is cooked. Rest tuna for 10 minutes, then slice into 5mm thick slices.

Blanch asparagus, uncovered, in a saucepan of boiling salted water for 1 minute, add sugar snap peas, blanch another 10 seconds, then drain and rinse under cold water. Pat dry with absorbent paper.

Combine chilli, green onions, blanched asparagus, sugar snap peas, salad leaves, roasted capsicum and half the herbs in a large bowl, add tamari dressing and toss gently. Divide salad mixture among bowls, top with sliced tuna and scatter with remaining herbs and flaked almonds.

SERVES 4 FOR LUNCH or 6 AS AN ENTREE

Tamari Dressing can be made 3 hours ahead.
Will keep, covered, at room temperature.

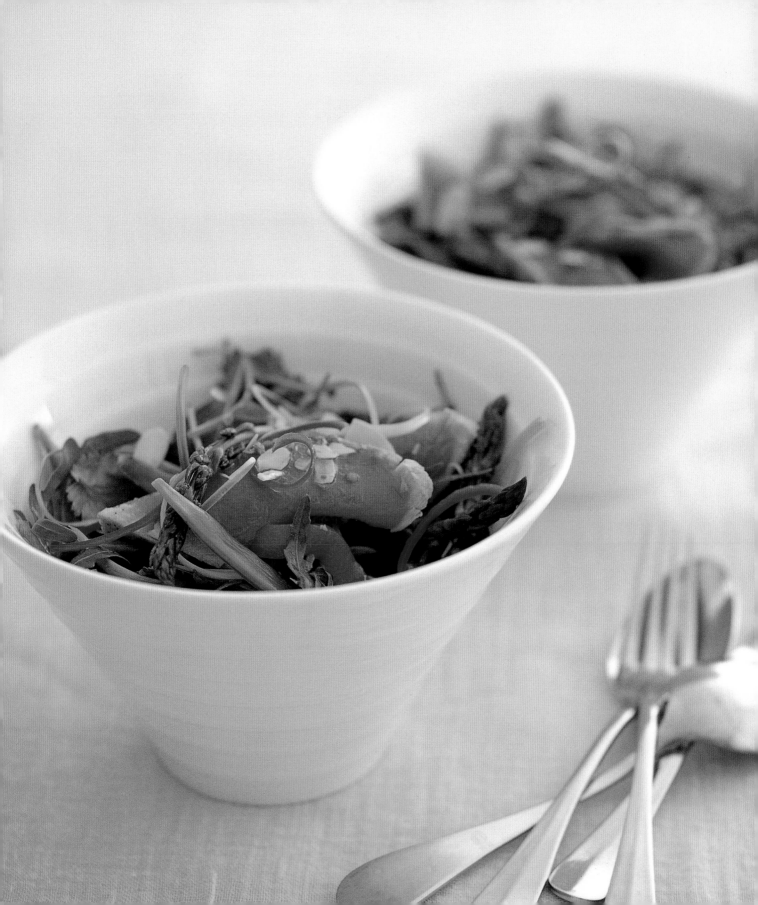

moreton bay bugs with soba noodles & green onions

Most fishmongers now sell shelled bug meat. If you can't get it, shell them yourself. You need to buy live bugs and place them in the freezer or an ice slurry to kill them kindly. Remove the heads. Using kitchen scissors, cut through the soft underside of the shell on both sides of the meat, peel the shell back, then pull out the meat. Use the shells for stock.

grapeseed oil

500 g Moreton Bay bug meat, halved
   lengthwise if large

2 large fresh red chillies, sliced, or to
   taste

2 cloves garlic, chopped

2 tsp grated ginger

8 green (spring) onions, sliced on the
   diagonal

grated rind and juice 1 lime

2 tbsp tamari

125 ml (1/2 cup) Chicken Stock
   (page 159)

250 g wheat-free soba noodles

sesame oil, to serve

Heat 1 tablespoon oil in a wok and stir-fry bug meat over high heat, in batches, until just browned and cooked. Remove from wok.

Add a little more oil to wok if necessary and stir-fry chilli, garlic, ginger and green onions over medium heat for 30 seconds. Add lime rind and juice, tamari and chicken stock and boil over high heat to reduce by half. Pour green onion mixture over bug meat and check seasoning, adding more lime juice, if necessary.

Cook noodles according to directions on packet, making sure not to overcook them. Toss bug mixture with noodles and serve drizzled with a little sesame oil.

SERVES 4

Recipe best made just before serving.

grilled polenta with tomato, red lentil & olive sauce

You can use instant polenta for this recipe – it only takes minutes to cook and is available from most supermarkets. The sauce is really delicious and is also suitable for serving over buckwheat or spelt pasta or with steamed rice and wilted spinach, or with our Spinach Gnocchi (page 136).

300 g polenta (yellow cornmeal)

olive oil

1/4 cup fresh baby basil leaves

TOMATO, RED LENTIL & OLIVE SAUCE

1 x 400 g can tomatoes

1 tbsp olive oil

100 g (1/2 cup) red lentils, rinsed

4 cloves garlic, chopped

1/4 tsp honey

80 g (1/2 cup) Kalamata olives, pitted
   and sliced

To make Tomato, Red Lentil & Olive Sauce, combine chopped tomatoes and their juice, oil, lentils, garlic, honey and 375 ml (1$\frac{1}{2}$ cups) water in a saucepan, season to taste and cook, uncovered, over medium heat for 15 minutes. Add olives and cook another 10 minutes or until lentils are tender and sauce is thick.

Bring 1.3 litres (5$\frac{1}{4}$ cups) water to the boil in a large saucepan, add salt to taste, reduce heat, add polenta in thin stream and stir well. Reduce heat to very low, cover and cook about 20 minutes, stirring occasionally with a whisk, until all the lumps are gone and polenta thickens and comes away from side of pan. Remove from heat, spoon onto a baking paper lined tray and shape into a 32 x 21 cm rectangle. When cold, cut into triangles and place on an oven tray.

Brush polenta with a little oil and grill on both sides until warm. Divide polenta among shallow bowls. Spoon Tomato, Red Lentil & Olive Sauce over and sprinkle with baby basil leaves.

SERVES 4–6

Polenta can be prepared a day ahead, Tomato, Red Lentil & Olive Sauce 3 days ahead. Keep, covered separately, in refrigerator.

avocado, roasted beetroot & lentil salad

Puy lentils are small dark blue-green lentils, originally from Le Puy in France, but now also grown in Australia. You can buy them from good delicatessens and food stores. Green lentils could be used instead but will give you a different flavour and texture.

2 large beetroot, trimmed and halved

100 g (1/2 cup) French green (Puy)
   lentils

1 tbsp extra virgin olive oil

1 tsp grated lemon rind

2 tbsp lemon juice

1 tbsp chopped fresh chives

1 tbsp chopped fresh tarragon

100 g watercress or rocket leaves

1 avocado, seeded, peeled and cut into
   2 cm pieces

extra fresh chives, cut into 4 cm
   lengths, to serve

Wrap beetroot in foil, place on an oven tray and roast at 200°C about 50–60 minutes or until tender when pierced with a knife. Remove foil and, when cool enough to handle, rub off skins and cut into wedges.

Cook lentils, uncovered, in simmering water about 20 minutes or until tender. Drain and rinse under cold water.

Combine oil, lemon rind, lemon juice and herbs and season to taste. Gently toss watercress or rocket with half the dressing. Toss lentils with remaining dressing.

Serve watercress or rocket leaves topped with avocado, lentils, beetroot and extra chives.

SERVES 4

Beetroot and lentils can be cooked a day ahead.
Will keep, covered separately, in refrigerator.

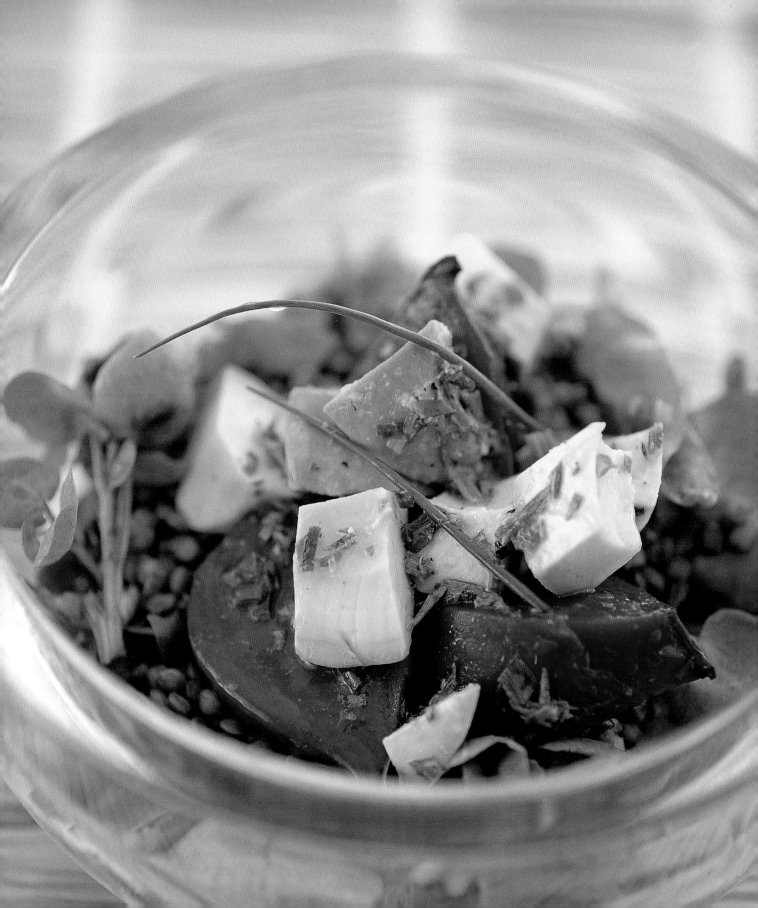

peter's favourite bean, rice & roasted carrot salad

A simple salad, this is great on its own, but also makes an excellent accompaniment to grilled lamb or chicken. Make sure you season this salad well otherwise the beans can be quite bland. Slice the carrots thinly – as they roast, their natural sugar will caramelise and give you a lovely intense flavour. This is a good one to pack up and take to work for lunch.

3 (450 g) carrots, thinly sliced crosswise

olive oil

1 tbsp red wine or balsamic vinegar

100 g (¹/₂ cup) dried borlotti beans,
   soaked in cold water overnight

200 g (1 cup) basmati rice

4 dried figs, coarsely chopped

40 g walnuts, lightly roasted, coarsely
   chopped

4 green (spring) onions, chopped

2 tbsp chopped fresh coriander

2 tbsp chopped fresh dill

4 large radicchio leaves

Yoghurt Dressing (page 164), to serve
   (optional)

Toss carrots with 1 tablespoon oil, spread on an oven tray and roast at 200°C for 25–30 minutes, or until golden and tender. Remove from oven, toss with vinegar and cool.

Cook drained borlotti beans, uncovered, in simmering water about 40–50 minutes or until tender, then drain.

Cook rice, uncovered, in simmering salted water for 10 minutes, drain and rinse under cold water.

Combine beans, rice, carrot mixture, figs, walnuts, green onions and herbs, stir in 1 tablespoon oil and season to taste. Place radicchio leaves on plates, top with salad and drizzle with Yoghurt Dressing, if using.

SERVES 4

Recipe can be made a day ahead.
Will keep, covered, in refrigerator.

green lentil & potato curry with coriander

This is wonderful served on its own, or with steamed rice for a more substantial meal, or as an excellent addition to a vegetarian buffet. It also works well as an accompaniment to grilled chicken. This is also an ideal dish to pack for lunch.

1 tbsp olive oil

2 onions, chopped

1 L (4 cups) Vegetable Stock (page 160) or water

500 g orange sweet potato, peeled and chopped into 3 cm pieces

500 g desiree potatoes, peeled and chopped into 3 cm pieces

200 g (1 cup) dried green lentils, rinsed

fresh coriander leaves, to serve

Yoghurt Dressing (page 164), to serve (optional)

SPICE PASTE

6 large fresh green chillies, seeded and chopped

80 ml (¹/₃ cup) lemon juice

6 cloves garlic, chopped

2 tsp grated ginger

1 cup fresh coriander (leaves and stalks), chopped

For Spice Paste, place all ingredients in a food processor and process until well combined.

Heat oil in a large saucepan and cook onion over low heat until soft, adding a little of the stock if onions are sticking to pan. Add spice paste and cook for 3 minutes or until aromatic. Add remaining ingredients and salt to taste and cook, covered, over low heat about 35 minutes until potato and lentils are soft and most of the stock has been absorbed. Check seasoning and serve warm topped with extra coriander leaves. Serve Yoghurt Dressing separately, if using.

SERVES 4–6

Recipe can be made a day ahead.
Will keep, covered, in refrigerator.

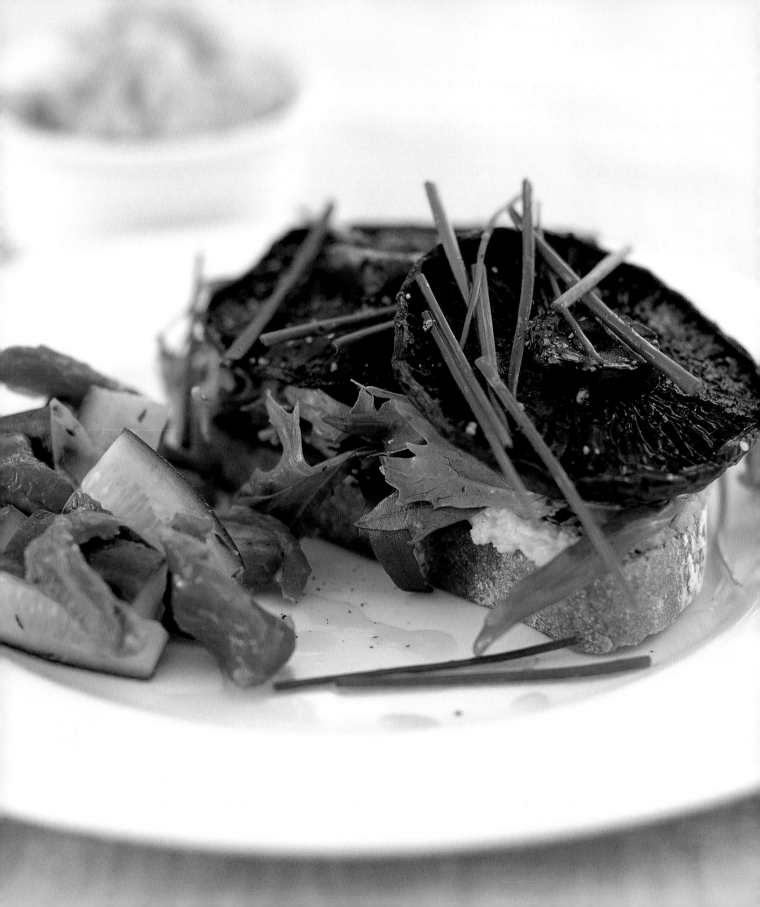

grilled mushrooms
& rocket on toast

We have used Swiss brown mushrooms here, but you could also use large flat field mushrooms. Basically, you are after nice big mushrooms with lots of flavour. Semi-dried tomatoes are now available from supermarkets, but in summer when tomatoes are plentiful it's great to make your own.

8 large Swiss brown mushrooms

extra virgin olive oil

1/2 cup Tahini & Almond Spread
  (page 165)

8 slices gluten-free, dark rye or
  spelt bread, toasted

100 g rocket leaves, trimmed

1 bunch fresh chives, cut into 4 cm
  lengths

100 g semi-dried tomatoes

2 Lebanese (small green) cucumbers,
  cut into wedges to match the
  tomatoes

1 tbsp lemon juice

Place mushrooms on an oven tray, brush with a little oil and season to taste. Place under a hot grill about 2 minutes until just cooked.

Spread Tahini & Almond Spread on toast and place 1–2 slices on each plate. Top toast with rocket and mushrooms and sprinkle with chives. Toss tomatoes with cucumbers and place to one side. Combine 1 tablespoon oil with lemon juice and drizzle around plate.

SERVES 4

Tahini & Almond Spread can be made 2 weeks ahead.
Will keep, covered, in refrigerator.

quinoa salad with slow-roasted mushrooms

Quinoa is an ancient high-protein grain and is available from health food stores. Cooking quinoa in stock gives it more flavour, but you can use water instead. We have **slow roasted** *the mushrooms here to intensify their flavour, but if you are pressed for time you could always grill them.*

500 ml (2 cups) Vegetable Stock (page 159) or water

190 g (1 cup) quinoa

1 stick celery, finely chopped

35 g (¼ cup) roasted hazelnuts, peeled and coarsely chopped

3 fresh dates, pitted and finely chopped

extra virgin olive oil

¼ preserved lemon, rinsed and flesh discarded

2 tbsp chopped fresh flat-leaf parsley

1 tbsp lemon juice

8 medium Swiss brown mushrooms

40 g snowpea sprouts, trimmed

Heat stock or water in a saucepan, add quinoa and cook, covered, over medium heat about 15 minutes or until quinoa is tender and stock is absorbed. Remove lid and stir over heat about 1 minute or until excess moisture is evaporated.

Combine quinoa, celery, hazelnuts and dates and toss well. Stir in 1 tablespoon oil, preserved lemon, parsley and lemon juice and season to taste.

Meanwhile place mushrooms on an oven tray, brush lightly with oil, season to taste and roast at 150°C for 20 minutes or until just tender.

Serve salad topped with mushrooms and snowpea sprouts and drizzle with a little extra oil.

SERVES 4

Best made just before serving.

vegetable & tofu rice paper rolls with dipping sauce

These rolls are fresh and crunchy and ideal for a picnic or to pass around at a party. For a seafood alternative, you could substitute the tofu with 200 g sashimi quality tuna. Rice paper is now found in some supermarkets or Asian food stores.

14 x 16 cm rice paper rounds

14 leaves fresh Vietnamese mint
  or mint

DIPPING SAUCE

2 tbsp wheat-free tamari sauce

2 tbsp lime juice

1/2 tsp sesame oil

1/2 large red chilli, sliced

1 tsp brown rice syrup

2 tsp sesame seeds, toasted

FILLING

200 g firm tofu

20 g dried shiitake mushrooms

25 g rice vermicelli noodles

1 tbsp coriander leaves

1 tbsp fresh Thai basil or basil leaves

1 tbsp fresh Vietnamese mint or
  mint leaves

2 green (spring) onions, cut into
  julienne

50 g daikon, peeled, cut into julienne

100 g carrot, peeled and cut into
  julienne

To make Dipping Sauce, combine all ingredients, season to taste and stand for 30 minutes for flavours to develop.

To make Filling, cut tofu into thin strips. Place mushrooms in a bowl, cover with 250 ml (1 cup) hot water and stand for 30 minutes, then strain through a fine sieve. Squeeze mushrooms to remove excess water. Remove and discard stems, then cut mushroom caps into 2 mm-thick slices.

Cook rice noodles according to directions on packet, then chop coarsely. Combine mushrooms, noodles and remaining ingredients, toss well and season to taste.

Soak rice paper in hot water, in batches until softened, then place on damp tea towels, covering with another damp tea towel as you work.

Place 1 mint leaf in centre of a rice paper round and top with 2–3 strips of tofu. Place about 1 tablespoon of filling on top. Roll up to form a parcel. Repeat process with remaining rice-paper rounds and ingredients. Serve Rice Paper Rolls with Dipping sauce.

MAKES 14

Dipping Sauce and rolls can be made 2 hours ahead.
Cover rolls with damp absorbent paper then plastic wrap
and keep at room temperature.

buckwheat pasta with broad beans, peas & cherry tomatoes

This is a very pretty dish and is lovely served in the spring when broad beans are plentiful. You will find buckwheat pasta at some supermarkets and health food stores. Be careful when cooking it as it can fall apart easily if overcooked.

250 g buckwheat pasta

500 g broad beans, podded

500 g peas, podded

1 tbsp olive oil

1 punnet cherry tomatoes

2 cloves garlic, chopped

1–2 large fresh red chillies, sliced,
  or to taste

90 g (¹/2 cup) baby olives, pitted

2 tbsp toasted pinenuts

¹/2 cup fresh basil leaves

Cook pasta, uncovered, in simmering salted water about 7 minutes or until al dente, drain and reserve 80 ml (¹/3 cup) cooking liquid.

Cook broad beans in simmering salted water, uncovered, for 3 minutes, then drain and rinse under cold water. Peel broad beans.

Cook peas in simmering salted water, uncovered, about 8 minutes or until tender. Drain and rinse under cold water.

Heat oil in a frying pan until hot and stir-fry tomatoes, garlic and chillies over high heat for 1 minute, then add reserved cooking liquid and heat through. Season tomato mixture to taste and toss with pasta. Stir in broad beans, peas, olives and pinenuts and serve sprinkled with basil.

SERVES 4–6

Best made just before serving.

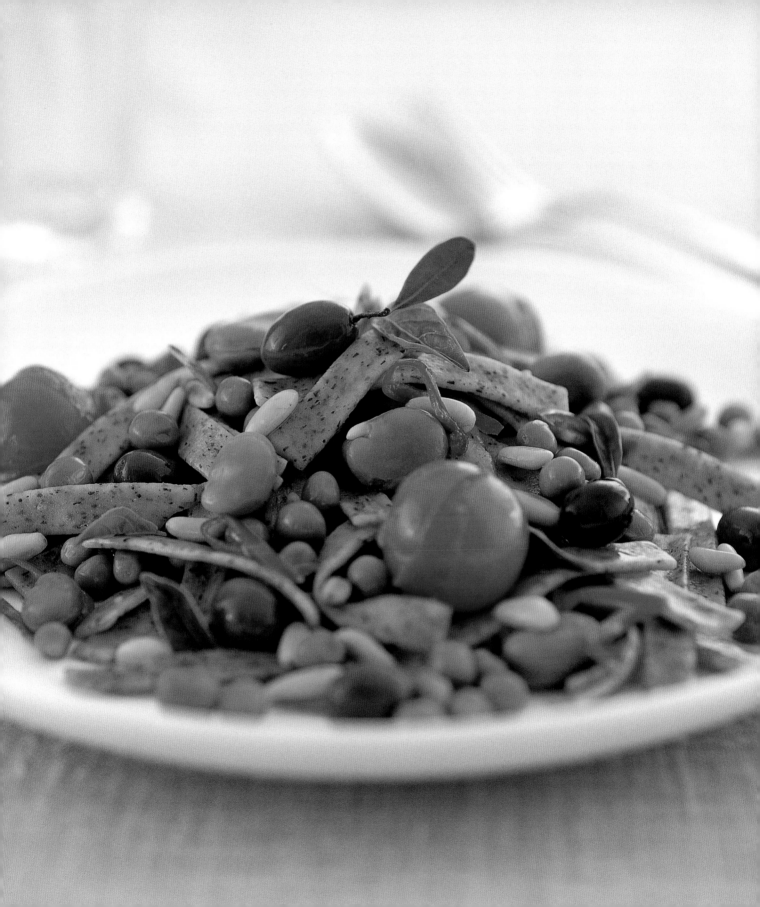

asparagus salad with poached egg & dukkah

This makes a great light lunch or entree. Dukkah is a delicious Mediterranean spice mix that is traditionally served with a dish of olive oil and bread for dipping. It is easy to make and also available from spice stores and specialist food stores.

16 cherry tomatoes, halved

24 spears asparagus, trimmed

extra virgin olive oil

2 tsp aged balsamic vinegar

1 tbsp white wine vinegar

4 eggs

50 g baby salad leaves

2 green (spring) onions, sliced on the
    diagonal

Dukkah (page 166), to serve

Place tomatoes, cut side up on an oven tray with asparagus, brush lightly with olive oil and season to taste. Roast at 200°C for 5 minutes or until asparagus is tender and browned. Remove from oven and drizzle tomatoes and asparagus with balsamic vinegar.

Bring a deep frying pan of salted water to the boil, add the white wine vinegar, then reduce to a gentle simmer. Carefully break 1 egg into a small bowl. Use a wooden spoon to swirl the water in pan to create a whirlpool. Tip egg into centre of whirlpool and cook about 4 minutes or until set on the outside. Using a slotted spoon remove from water and place in a dish of cold water until ready to use. Repeat with remaing eggs.

Divide salad leaves among plates, top with green onions, tomatoes and asparagus and their dressing and poached egg. Serve sprinkled with Dukkah.

SERVES 4

Best made just before serving.

roasted vegetables with fennel & white bean puree

Try roasting sliced pumpkin, halved carrots, mushrooms or beetroot. If you can't get quail eggs, serve with halved boiled free-range eggs. This puree is fabulous served with crudités, or spread on rye bread and topped with smoked trout and sprigs of dill.

1 small eggplant, sliced crosswise into
   1 cm thick slices

2 zucchini, sliced lengthwise into 5 mm
   thick slices

300 g orange sweet potato, peeled,
   sliced crosswise into 1 cm thick slices

12 spears asparagus, trimmed

2 tbsp extra virgin olive oil

12 quail eggs

1 Roasted Capsicum (page 163)

FENNEL & WHITE BEAN PUREE

1 knob (head) garlic

100 g (1/2 cup) dried cannellini beans,
   soaked in cold water overnight

1 dried bay leaf

350 g bulb fennel, trimmed, cored and
   chopped

80 ml (1/3 cup) Vegetable Stock
   (page 159) or water

1 tbsp olive oil

To make Fennel & White Bean Puree, cover garlic with foil, place on an oven tray and roast at 200°C about 30 minutes or until garlic cloves are tender when pierced with a knife. Cool, then squeeze garlic from cloves.

Combine drained beans and bay leaf in a saucepan, cover with water and bring to the boil. Reduce heat and simmer, uncovered, about 30 minutes or until beans are tender. Drain and discard bay leaf.

Meanwhile combine fennel, stock or water and oil in a saucepan, bring to the boil and simmer, covered, over low heat about 30 minutes or until fennel is tender. Combine warm fennel mixture, warm beans and garlic paste in a food processor or hand-held blender and process until smooth, then season to taste.

Place eggplant, zucchini, sweet potato and asparagus in a large bowl and toss with oil. Place eggplant and zucchini on one oven tray and sweet potato and asparagus on another. Roast at 200°C for 10 minutes, then remove asparagus and turn remaining vegetables over. Roast another 25 minutes, then remove eggplant and zucchini. Cook sweet potato another 10 minutes until tender and browned.

Add quail eggs to simmering water and cook, uncovered, for 3 minutes. Drain, rinse under cold water and peel.

Place roasted vegetables in rows on a large platter with the quail eggs and serve with a bowl of Fennel & White Bean Puree.

SERVES 4 FOR LUNCH or 8 AS PART OF AN ANTIPASTO PLATTER

Makes about 500 ml (2 cups) puree.

Puree can be made 3 days ahead. Will keep, covered, in refrigerator.

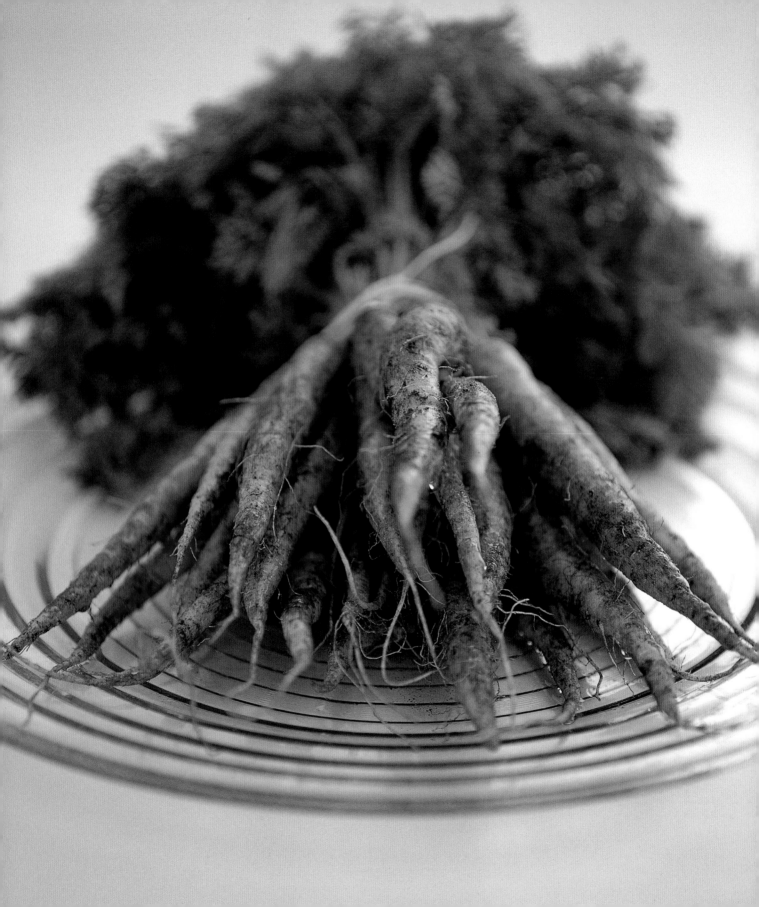

three dips with toast & crudités

This is very versatile and can be served for lunch with a green salad, as an entree, or at a party or for a snack. The dips also make good side dishes for other recipes and are all excellent served with our Roasted Vegetables (page 89).

1 cup Hummus (page 165)

2 carrots, peeled and cut into sticks

2 sticks celery, cut into sticks

1 red capsicum, cut into sticks

1 zucchini, cut into sticks

1 witlof, leaves separated

gluten-free, rye or spelt bread, toasted,
  or Spiced Bran Crackers (page 35)

GREEN OLIVE & LENTIL DIP

100 g (1/2 cup) dried green lentils,
  rinsed

80 g (1/2 cup) green olives, pitted

2 tsp drained capers

2 tbsp lemon juice

1 clove garlic, chopped

1 tbsp fresh oregano leaves

1 tbp olive oil

MUSHROOM PÂTÉ

1 tbsp olive oil

250 g flat mushrooms, chopped

2 cloves garlic, chopped

1 tbsp lemon juice

30 g soft tofu, chopped

To make Green Olive & Lentil Dip, cook lentils, uncovered, in simmering water about 30 minutes or until tender, then drain and rinse under cold water. Combine lentils and remaining ingredients in a food processor and process until smooth, then season to taste.

To make Mushroom Pâté, heat olive oil in a large non-stick frying pan and stir-fry mushrooms over high heat until just wilted. Add garlic and lemon juice and stir-fry until mushroom juices have evaporated. Combine mushroom mixture and tofu in a food processor and process until smooth, then season to taste.

Serve Green Olive & Lentil Dip, Mushroom Pâté and Hummus with crudités and toasted bread or spiced bran crackers.

SERVES 10 AS AN APPETISER or 6 FOR LUNCH

Makes about 1 1/4 cups green olive & lentil dip

Makes about 1 1/4 cups mushroom pâté

Green Olive & Lentil Dip will keep, covered, in refrigerator for 3 days.

Mushroom Pâté will keep, covered, in refrigerator for 3 days.

Hummus will keep, covered, in refrigerator for 5 days.

stuffed zucchini flowers with tomato & red onion salsa

Served as a light lunch or as an entree, the success of this recipe depends on the freshness of the zucchini flowers. They need to be picked the day before so that the flower is crisp and firm, rather than wilted. That way they retain their shape and texture when they are steamed.

160 g soft tofu, drained

1 clove garlic, crushed

1 tbsp pinenuts, toasted and chopped

2 tbsp finely chopped mixed fresh
herbs, including basil, tarragon and
chives

12 zucchini flowers, with baby zucchini
attached

TOMATO & RED ONION SALSA

3 vine-ripened tomatoes, seeded and
chopped

1/4 small red (Spanish) onion, finely
chopped

1 tsp fresh thyme leaves

1 tbsp lemon juice

1 tbsp olive oil

To make Tomato & Red Onion Salsa, combine all ingredients and season to taste.

Place tofu in a bowl and mash with a fork until smooth. Stir in garlic, pinenuts and herbs and season to taste.

Gently prise open 1 zucchini flower and using a teaspoon, fill centre with tofu mixture. Twist blossom end to seal. Repeat with remaining flowers and filling. Place zucchini flowers, in batches, in a steaming basket lined with baking paper and place basket over a pan of simmering water. Cover basket with a lid and steam about 3 minutes or until zucchini are just tender when pierced with a knife.

Divide warm zucchini flowers among plates and serve immediately with Tomato & Red Onion Salsa.

SERVES 4

Tomato & Red Onion Salsa can be made 2 hours ahead.
Will keep, covered, at room temperature.

taking lunch to work

Many of the recipes in this chapter travel well and are ideal to take to work for lunch to be reheated or eaten as they are, or they can be taken on a picnic. Also, if you have leftovers from dinner, especially vegetables, then they can often become the next day's lunch too. If you are taking a salad, we suggest you leave the dressing separate, to add just before serving.

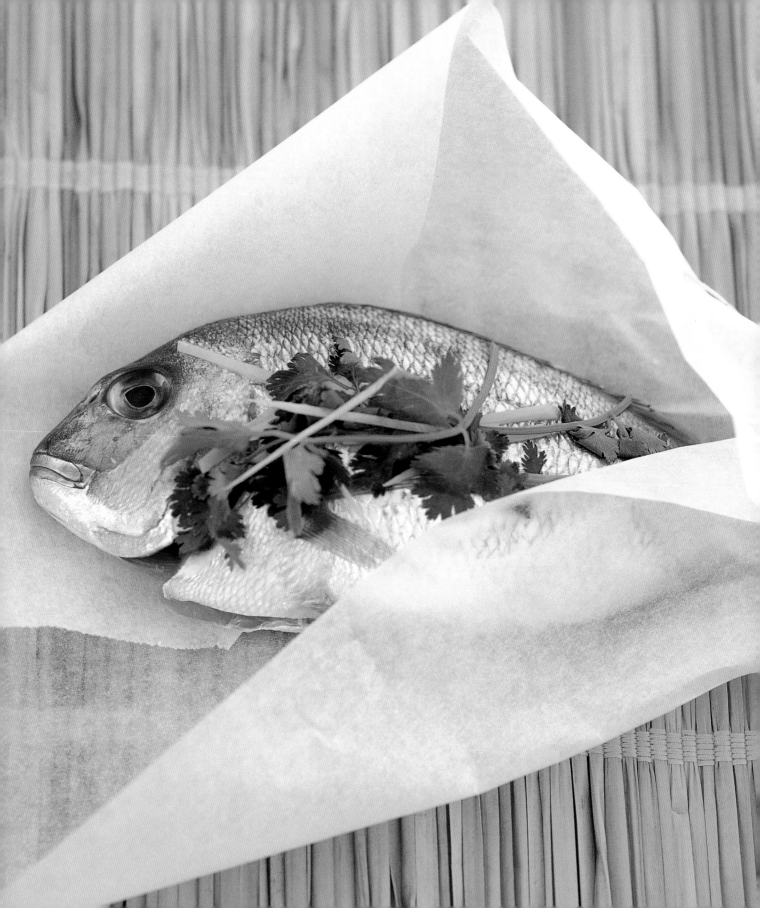

dinner

KATHY: The evening meal is my favourite, relaxing with my husband Peter, discussing the day over a plate of good food. It's never a chore to cook and when I am detoxing, I usually have so much more energy, I whip around the kitchen even faster. I eat a large variety of food over a week, including plenty of vegetables and leafy greens and lots of seafood. The only dish I really miss when I am detoxing is roast chicken (I can't bear to forego the crisp skin) but the Asian-style Poached Chicken (page 96) is so good it helps to fill the gap. If I go out to eat when I'm detoxing, I look for seafood on the menu.

JAN: My partner Gavin is as passionate about food as I am. We often cook our meals together (quite harmoniously) with one of us taking the role of 'head chef' while the other is 'kitchen hand'. We really enjoy sitting down at the table to enjoy the fruits of our labour together. Our meals are generally so healthy that doing a detox might mean foregoing that fabulous red or white wine, pasta or couscous – the rest is easy. Whether detoxing or not, vegetables are abundant in our dinner meals.

These dishes are a little more substantial than the recipes in the lunch chapter and some require a bit more preparation, but essentially they are stylish and based on flavour and freshness.

One of the key factors in maintaining a successful detox is not to feel deprived, so it's a good idea to write a simple menu plan for the week. That way, you know you have delicious meals to look forward to. This will also help with the shopping. Make sure you have a stock of dry goods such as rice, polenta, noodles and quinoa on hand and where possible shop daily for fresh ingredients. In the evening, make yourself a fresh juice to sip on while you are preparing dinner.

We have created dishes that are so appetising, the whole family will love them even if they are not detoxing. If you are dining out, it's easy – order simple dishes such as grilled fish or chicken with side dishes of salad (ask for it without the dressing) and vegetables, or choose a restaurant that has a large selection of vegetarian dishes. Asian-style restaurants, particularly Vietnamese, Indian or Japanese restaurants, are a good choice.

With our list of stylish recipes to hand, it's also easy to entertain while you are detoxing. Your friends will love the food and you will find that many of these recipes will become standbys whether you are detoxing or not.

asian-style poached chicken with rice noodles

Considering the short cooking time of the chicken, it always amazes us how perfectly it cooks, delivering snowy white and moist flesh each time. Here we serve the chicken with noodles, but the more traditional accompaniment is rice, cooked in the stock, with the remaining stock served as a broth. You can remove the skin from the chicken before serving if you like.

2 cm piece ginger, peeled and sliced

2 star anise

2 cloves garlic, halved

1 onion, halved

2 fresh coriander roots

1.8 kg chicken

15 g dried shiitake mushrooms, soaked in hot water for 30 minutes

100 g rice vermicelli noodles

1 tbsp light olive oil

8 green (spring) onions, sliced on the diagonal

4 baby bok choy, trimmed and leaves separated

1/2 cup fresh coriander leaves

1/2 cup fresh mint leaves

soy sauce or wheat-free tamari sauce and sesame oil, to taste

CHILLI SAUCE

4 large fresh red chillies, chopped

2 cloves garlic, chopped

juice from 2 limes

1 tsp grated ginger

To make Chilli Sauce, combine all ingredients in a mortar and pound with a pestle until smooth, then season to taste with salt. Alternatively combine all ingredients in a small food processor and process until smooth.

Place 4 litres (16 cups) water in a large stockpot, add ginger, star anise, garlic, onion, coriander roots and 2 teaspoons salt and bring to the boil. Tie chicken with string to form a loop to hold it, rub all over with salt. Lower into simmering stock for 30 seconds, then remove. Repeat this 3 times.

Return chicken to pot and simmer, uncovered, over gentle heat for 15 minutes. Turn off heat, cover with a lid and stand 45 minutes. Remove chicken from stock and plunge into cold water for 1 hour. Remove and cut into serving pieces. Strain stock through a muslin-lined sieve and discard solids. Remove fat from surface and reserve stock.

Meanwhile, drain shiitake mushrooms and slice thinly. Cook noodles according to directions on packet. Heat oil in a wok and stir-fry mushrooms and half the green onions for 1 minute, then add bok choy and stir-fry until just wilted. Add 250 ml (1 cup) reserved stock and heat through, then stir in half the herbs and drained noodles. Reserve remaining stock for another use.

Serve noodle mixture in warm bowls topped with chicken, remaining green onions and herbs, then drizzle with a little soy sauce or tamari and sesame oil to taste. Serve Chilli Sauce separately.

SERVES 4

Chilli Sauce can be made a day ahead. Will keep, covered, in refrigerator.

braised chicken
with wild rice

The addition of a little vinegar to the braising liquid for this dish adds a lovely sharp tangy bite. If you suffer from recurrent thrush, cystitis or tinea then it would be best to omit the vinegar and deglaze the pan with a little stock or water. If you can't get wild rice, serve this dish with basmati rice cooked according to directions on the packet.

olive oil

1 onion, chopped

400 ml Chicken Stock (page 159)

2–3 tbsp white wine vinegar, or to taste

2 cloves garlic, chopped

1 small fresh red chilli, seeded, chopped

4 large vine-ripened tomatoes, peeled, seeded and chopped

4 skinless chicken breast fillets, halved crosswise

2 tbsp shredded fresh basil

90 g (1/2 cup) wild rice

2 tsp butter

200 g baby beans, trimmed

4 zucchini, cut into batons

Heat 1 tablespoon oil in a large heavy-based casserole and cook onion over low heat until soft, adding a little stock if onion is sticking to pan. Add vinegar to deglaze pan, then add garlic, chilli and tomatoes and cook, uncovered, over high heat until tomatoes are thick and pulpy. Add stock, bring to the boil and simmer, uncovered, until sauce is reduced by half, then season to taste.

Brush chicken with a little olive oil and brown in a non-stick pan over high heat. Add chicken pieces to tomato mixture and cook, covered, over low heat about 20 minutes or until chicken is just cooked, then stir in basil.

Meanwhile cook wild rice, uncovered, in simmering salted water about 20 minutes, or until tender. Drain, stir in butter and season to taste. Steam beans and zucchini until tender.

Spoon rice into shallow bowls, top with chicken mixture and serve beans and zucchini to one side.

SERVES 4

Chicken can be braised a day ahead, then reheated gently.
Will keep, covered, in refrigerator.

chicken & vegetable stew with capsicum & walnut pistou

This dish is light and fresh and perfect for summer days as well as cooler weather. The pistou is also delightful spread on gluten-free bread or crispbread and topped with rocket leaves, avocado and grilled mushrooms, or served with grilled fish.

100 g (1/2 cup) dried cannellini beans, soaked overnight in cold water

1 tbsp olive oil

1 leek, white part only, trimmed and sliced into 1 cm thick slices

1 baby fennel bulb, trimmed, cored and chopped

1 stick celery, coarsely chopped

1.5 L (6 cups) Chicken Stock (page 159), reduced to 1 L

2 cloves garlic, chopped

1 small fresh red chilli, seeded and chopped

4 vine-ripened tomatoes, peeled, seeded and chopped

2 desiree potatoes, peeled and cut into 2 cm pieces

1/2 Poached Chicken, (page 161), skinned, flesh torn into bite-sized pieces

thyme sprigs, to serve

CAPSICUM & WALNUT PISTOU

1 Roasted Capsicum (page 163)

2 cloves garlic, chopped

1 small fresh red chilli, seeded and chopped

50 g walnuts, lightly roasted

To make Capsicum & Walnut Pistou, combine capsicum and any of its roasting juices, garlic, chilli and walnuts in a food processor and process until smooth, then season to taste with salt.

Cook drained beans, uncovered, in simmering water about 30 minutes or until just tender, then drain.

Heat olive oil in a large heavy-based saucepan and cook leek, fennel and celery, covered, over low heat until soft, adding a little stock if vegetables are sticking to pan. Add garlic, chilli and tomatoes and cook over high heat until tomatoes are soft and pulpy. Add potatoes and stock and simmer, uncovered, over medium heat until potatoes are tender. Add beans and cook another 5 minutes. Add chicken and stir in one third of the Capsicum & Walnut Pistou. Season to taste and simmer gently about 5 minutes or until chicken is heated through.

Ladle chicken and vegetable stew into warm bowls, sprinkle with a few sprigs of thyme and serve remaining Capsicum & Walnut Pistou separately.

SERVES 4

Makes about 250 ml (1 cup) pistou

Will keep, covered, in refrigerator for 3 days.

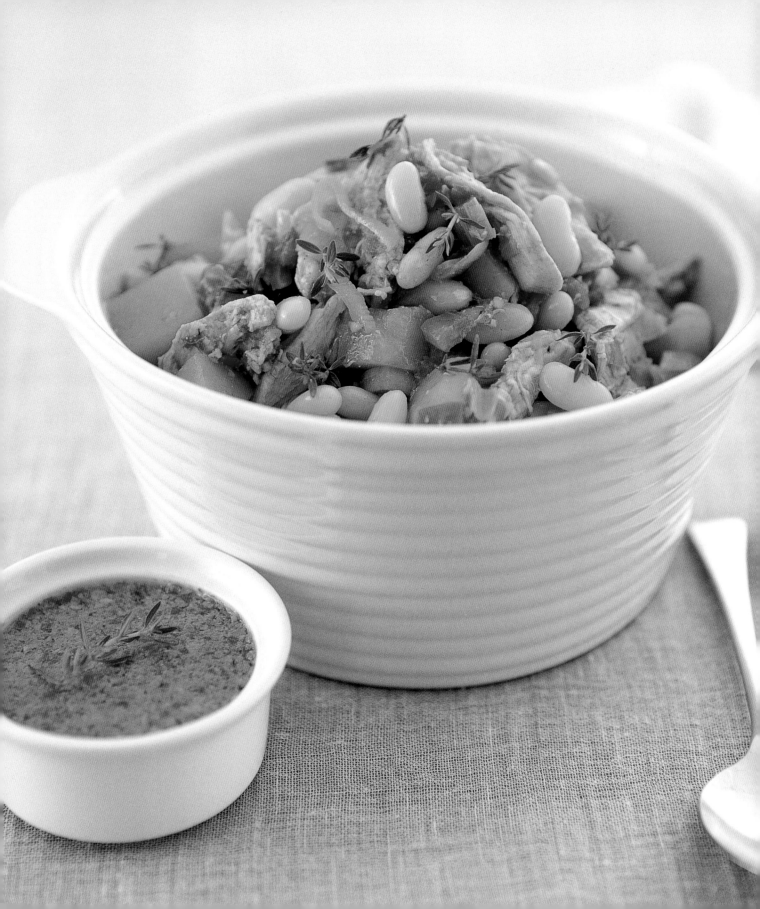

chicken & bean paella

Contrary to popular belief, the Spanish rarely mix meat and seafood in their paella. We love this version, using chicken and both dried and fresh beans. It is traditional in Spain to serve paella with alioli (the Spanish version of garlic mayonnaise), so if you want to add a little drizzle of Light Mayonnaise do so.

100 g (^{1}/2 cup) dried cannellini beans, soaked in cold water overnight

1 tbsp olive oil

3 chicken breast fillets, halved crosswise

1 onion, chopped

1 L (4 cups) hot Chicken Stock (page 159), approximately

3 cloves garlic, chopped

5 large vine-ripened tomatoes, peeled, seeded, chopped

^{1}/2 tsp sweet paprika

2 dried bay leaves

^{1}/2 tsp saffron threads, soaked in 1 tbsp hot water 10 minutes

300 g (1^1/2 cups) Calasparra or arborio rice

150 g flat roman beans, trimmed and cut into 4 cm lengths

Light Mayonnaise (page 164), to serve (optional)

Leafy Green Salad (page 161), to serve

Cook drained cannellini beans in simmering water about 30 minutes, or until tender. Drain.

Heat oil in a 34 cm paella pan and cook chicken pieces in batches over high heat until just browned, then remove from pan. Add onion and cook over low heat until soft, adding a little stock if onion is sticking to pan. Add garlic, tomatoes, paprika, bay leaves and saffron mixture and cook over high heat until tomatoes are pulpy. Add rice and stir to coat with mixture. Add 250 ml (1 cup) hot stock and cook over high heat for 5 minutes to create a crust on bottom of pan. Add ^{3}/4 of remaining stock, chicken and both beans and season to taste. Do not stir. Cook, uncovered, over medium heat another 20 minutes or until chicken is tender, rice is cooked and stock has been absorbed, adding more stock if necessary. The rice should be quite dry. Remove from heat and cover with a clean tea towel for 10 minutes. Serve with Light Mayonnaise, if using, and Leafy Green Salad.

SERVES 4–6

Best made just before serving.

chargrilled quail with buckwheat noodles

Buckwheat noodles are delicious but quite fragile, so it's important not to overcook them. There are various brands on the market, so check the cooking directions for each and make sure the brand you buy is wheat-free. For a vegetarian alternative you could use vegetable stock and substitute chargrilled tofu for the quail.

1 L (4 cups) Chicken Stock (page 159)

2 stalks fresh lemongrass, trimmed and bruised

2 star anise

4 cloves garlic

6 slices ginger

1 carrot, peeled and cut into julienne

100 g snowpeas, cut into julienne

1 baby bok choy, trimmed and shredded lengthwise

250 g buckwheat noodles

4 large quail, halved and backbone removed

olive oil

fresh mint and coriander leaves, shredded, to serve

DRESSING

1 large fresh red chilli, sliced

1 tsp sesame oil

1 tbsp wheat-free tamari sauce

1 tbsp shaohsing wine vinegar

1/4 tsp honey, or to taste

To make Dressing, combine all ingredients and stand for 30 minutes for flavours to develop.

Combine stock, lemongrass, star anise, garlic and ginger in a saucepan and cook, uncovered, over high heat until reduced by half. Strain stock and discard solids.

Combine carrots, snowpeas and bok choy in a bowl, pour boiling water over, then drain, rinse under cold water and drain again.

Cook noodles according to directions on packet. Combine noodles and vegetables in a bowl and toss gently.

Meanwhile, brush quail lightly with oil and chargrill about 3 minutes each side for pink or until cooked to your liking.

Divide noodle mixture among shallow bowls and pour hot stock over. Top with quail and herbs and drizzle with dressing.

SERVES 4

Dressing can be made 3 hours ahead.
Will keep, covered, at room temperature.

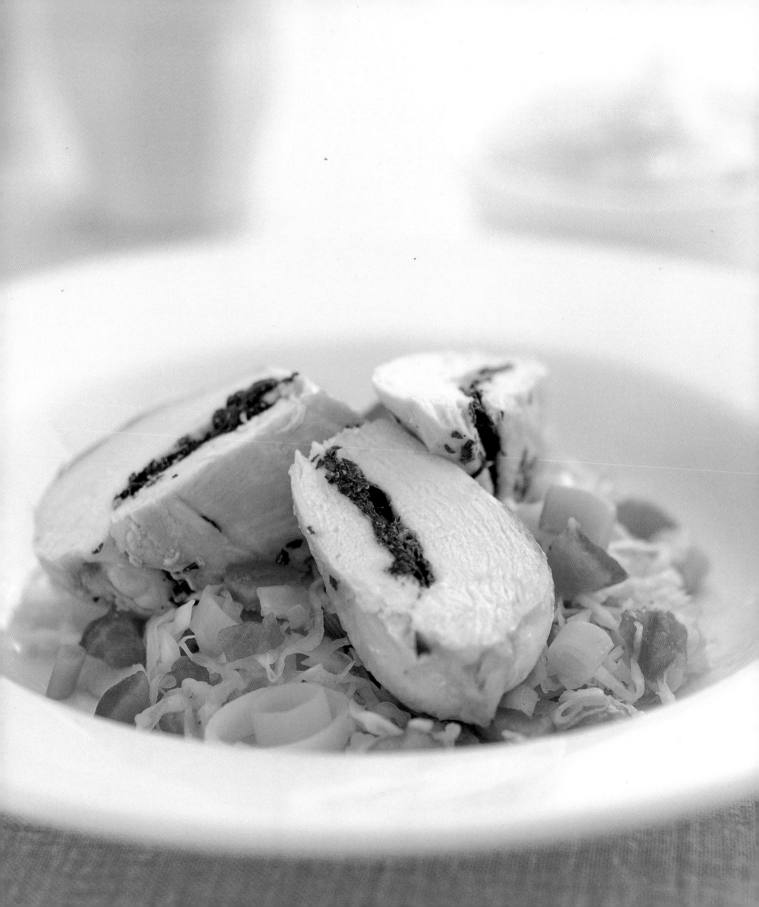

roasted chicken breast with braised cabbage & mash

We have removed the tenderloin from the breast fillets for this dish, to reduce the cooking time and to ensure that they don't dry out in the oven without the skin. Reserve the tenderloins for another dish – they could be used for our Chicken Kebabs with Baby Spinach & Pomegranate Salad (page 56).

4 skinless chicken breast fillets,
  tenderloin removed

1/4 cup chopped mixed herbs, including
  basil, mint, coriander, flat-leaf parsley

2 cloves garlic, finely chopped

2 tsp grated lemon rind

olive oil

1 leek, trimmed and sliced 1 cm thick
  crosswise

450 g (about 1/4) Savoy cabbage,
  shredded

2 vine-ripened tomatoes, peeled,
  seeded, chopped

Garlic Mash (page 160), to serve

Cut a pocket in the side of each chicken breast. Combine herbs, garlic and lemon rind, season to taste and divide among pockets. Secure with a toothpick.

Heat 1 tablespoon oil in a non-stick frying pan and cook chicken over high heat on both sides until well browned. Place on an oven tray and roast at 200°C about 15–20 minutes or until cooked. Remove from oven and rest in a warm place for 10 minutes. Remove toothpicks.

Meanwhile, heat 1 tablespoon oil in a saucepan and cook leek over low heat until soft. Add cabbage, season to taste and cook, covered, over medium heat, stirring occasionally, until cabbage is wilted, then stir in tomato and cook another 2 minutes.

Slice each chicken breast crosswise into three pieces and serve on a bed of wilted cabbage. Serve mash separately.

SERVES 4

Best made just before serving.

chargrilled lamb backstrap with caper & olive salsa

We chargrill over a grill pan across one or two burners on the top of the stove. That way, the vegetables, meat, chicken or seafood never comes into contact with a naked flame and you are able to control the charring effect. Brown the meat first, then turn down the heat and cook until it's done to your liking. Don't overbrown the meat.

1 tbsp chopped fresh rosemary

2 cloves garlic, chopped

grated rind and juice of 1 lemon

1 tbsp olive oil

750 g lamb backstraps (eye of loin)

basmati rice, steamed according to
   directions on packet, or Garlic Mash
   (page 160), to serve

Roasted Beetroot & Rocket Salad
   (page 162), to serve

CAPER & OLIVE SALSA

1/2 cup mixed chopped fresh herbs,
   including mint, basil, coriander

1 eschallot, finely chopped

1 tbsp capers, drained and chopped

40 g (1/4 cup) Kalamata olives, pitted
   and chopped

2 tbsp lemon juice

1 tbsp olive oil

To make Caper & Olive Salsa, combine all ingredients and season to taste.

Combine rosemary, garlic, lemon rind and juice and oil. Toss lamb in marinade and stand at room temperature for 1 hour.

Chargrill lamb or cook under a hot grill about 5 minutes on each side for pink lamb or until cooked to your liking. Remove lamb from heat and rest, loosely covered with foil, in a warm place for 10 minutes.

Slice lamb on the diagonal and serve on a bed of steamed rice or Garlic Mash. Top with Caper & Olive Salsa and serve with Roasted Beetroot & Rocket Salad.

SERVES 4

Caper & Olive Salsa can be made 3 hours ahead.
Will keep, covered, at room temperature.

lamb cutlets with white bean & cauliflower puree

White beans are very nutritious, great carriers of flavour and form a smooth creamy puree when processed. You can add all sorts of flavours to the puree, including cooked mushrooms or roasted garlic or braised fennel. Here, we add some roasted cauliflower to team with lamb cutlets. You could also use the puree as a dip with our Spiced Bran Crackers (page 35).

400 g baby beans, trimmed

olive oil

1 eschallot, finely chopped

12 cherry tomatoes, halved

12 lamb cutlets, trimmed of fat

WHITE BEAN AND CAULIFLOWER PUREE

100 g ($\frac{1}{2}$ cup) cannellini beans, soaked in cold water overnight

$\frac{1}{2}$ cauliflower, trimmed and cut into florets

$\frac{1}{4}$ cup lemon juice

GREMOLATA

2 cloves garlic, finely chopped

2 tbsp finely chopped fresh flat-leaf parsley

2 tsp grated lemon rind

To make White Bean and Cauliflower Puree, cook drained cannellini beans, uncovered, in simmering water about 30 minutes or until tender. Drain and reserve cooking liquid.

Place cauliflower on an oven tray, brush with a little oil and roast at 200°C about 20 minutes or until cauliflower is browned on edges and tender. Combine beans and cauliflower in a food processor, add lemon juice and 60 ml ($\frac{1}{4}$ cup) reserved cooking liquid and process until smooth, adding more cooking liquid if necessary, to form a smooth puree. Season to taste.

Cook baby beans in simmering salted water until tender, then drain and rinse under cold water. Heat 1 tablespoon oil in same saucepan, add eschallot and tomatoes and cook over high heat for 1 minute. Return beans to pan and toss to combine, then season to taste.

To make Gremolata, combine all ingredients and season to taste.

Meanwhile, brush cutlets with a little oil and pan fry in a non-stick frying pan on both sides until tender.

Spread White Bean and Cauliflower Puree on plates, top with green bean mixture and cutlets and spoon Gremolata over.

SERVES 4

Gremolata can be made 3 hours ahead.
Will keep, covered, at room temperature.

duck, sweet corn & herb risotto

A few years ago, you couldn't find decent duck in Australia, but now we have a regular supply of firm flavoursome birds. As duck is very fatty, you will need to trim the skin and fat off the breasts before you cook them. If you are not in detox mode and want to leave it on, score the skin and cook, skin side down, in a non-stick pan for about 2 minutes until the skin is crisp and browned, then roast as below.

2 corn cobs

2 zucchini, chopped

olive oil

1 onion, chopped

2 cloves garlic, chopped

300 g (1½ cups) arborio rice

1 L (4 cups) Chicken Stock (page 159),
    approximately

¼ cup fresh basil leaves

¼ cup fresh coriander leaves

4 duck breasts, skin removed

Leafy Green Salad (page 161), to serve

Using a small serrated knife, remove kernels from corn cob. Place corn kernels and zucchini on an oven tray, brush with a little oil and roast at 200°C about 20 minutes or until tender and browned. Remove from oven and set aside.

Heat 1 tablespoon oil in a saucepan and cook onion over low heat until soft. Add garlic and rice and stir to coat in oil and toast lightly. Have stock simmering in another pan.

Add 250 ml (1 cup) stock to rice mixture and stir over low to medium heat until stock is absorbed. Add remaining stock 125 ml (½ cup) at a time and stir continuously, allowing each addition to be absorbed before adding the next, until rice is just tender (al dente). Add corn, zucchini and half the herbs with last addition of stock and season to taste. Remove from heat and cover with a lid for 5 minutes.

Meanwhile, brush duck breasts with a little olive oil and cook in a non-stick frying pan over high until browned on both sides. Transfer to an oven tray and roast at 200°C for 7 minutes for pink. Rest in a warm place for 10 minutes, before slicing on the diagonal.

Serve risotto topped with sliced duck and remaining herbs. Serve with Leafy Green Salad.

SERVES 4

Best made just before serving.

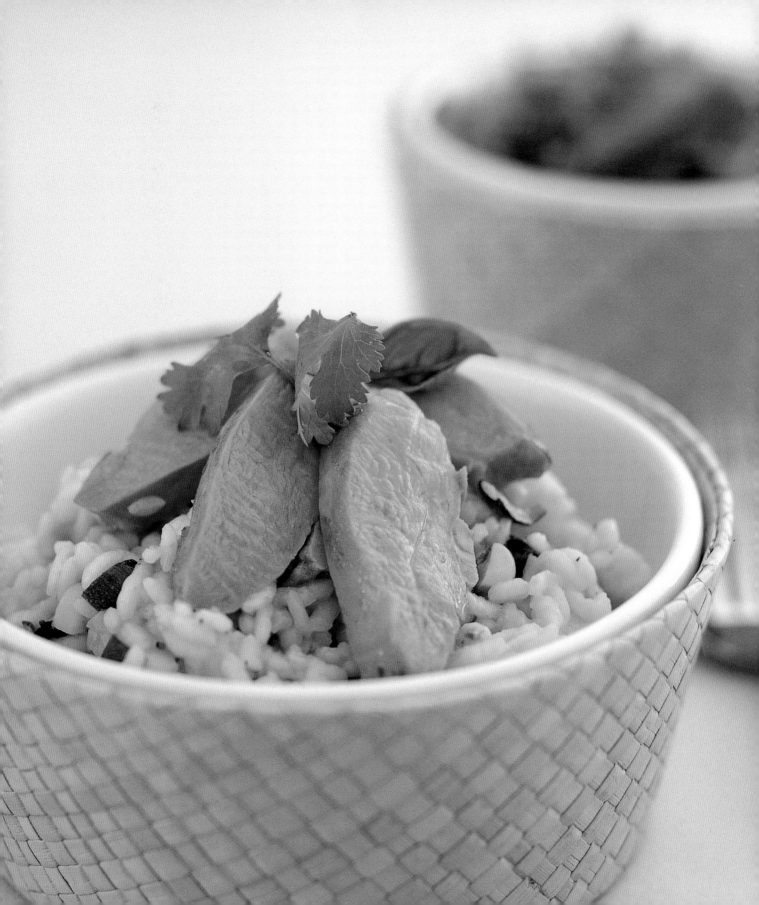

roasted venison with soft polenta & mushroom sauce

Vension and mushrooms both have earthy flavours and are heavenly together. Venison is a rich meat with a wonderful coarse texture, very low in fat and a good source of iron. Because of the low fat content, it's best served rare to medium so that it's not dry.

800 g venison topside

olive oil

400 g Swiss brown mushrooms, chopped

60 ml (¼ cup) Chicken Stock (page 159)

2 cloves garlic, chopped

2 tbsp verjuice or lemon juice

1 bunch English spinach, trimmed and wilted, to serve

1 bunch broccolini, trimmed and steamed, to serve

SOFT POLENTA

1.5 L (6 cups) Chicken Stock (page 159)

150 g polenta (yellow cornmeal)

To make Soft Polenta, bring chicken stock to the boil and whisk in polenta and salt to taste. Cook polenta over lowest heat, stirring regularly with a whisk about 30 minutes or until soft. The polenta should be soft and flowing, if it is too stiff add a little boiling water.

Brush venison with a little oil. Heat a non-stick frying pan and cook venison over high heat until lightly browned. Transfer to an oven tray and roast at 200°C for 30 minutes for rare. Reserve frying pan. Remove venison from oven, cover loosely with foil and rest in a warm place for 10 minutes before slicing on the diagonal.

Meanwhile, heat 1 tablespoon oil in reserved frying pan, add mushrooms and stock and cook over high heat until mushrooms have wilted. Add garlic and verjuice or lemon juice and cook over medium heat until juices are reduced, then season to taste.

Spoon polenta into bowls, top with spinach, broccolini, sliced venison and mushrooms.

SERVES 4

Best made just before serving.

slow roasted lamb with roasted vegetables

Cooking lamb at a low temperature for a longer period of time ensures that it is full of flavour and very juicy, but still remains pink in the centre. Make sure you rest the lamb well before carving, so the juices set. This recipe serves four generously and could stretch to six.

4 large cloves of garlic, peeled

1 teaspoon cumin seeds

1 teaspoon fennel seeds

2 teaspoons chopped thyme

olive oil

1.8 kg leg of lamb, trimmed of fat

2 cups Chicken Stock (page 159)

2 carrots, peeled and quartered
 lengthwise

2 parsnips, peeled and quartered
 lengthwise

2 leeks, white part only, cut crosswise
 into 4

2 baby bulbs fennel, trimmed and
 quartered

1 cup flat-leaf parsley leaves

35g (¼ cup) currants, soaked in warm
 water for 10 minutes, then drained

Combine garlic, cumin and fennel seeds, thyme and a good pinch of salt in a mortar and pound with a pestle until a paste forms. Stir in 1 tablespoon olive oil. Make small incisions over lamb and push half the paste mixture into the incisions, then rub the remaining mixture over lamb. Cover and refrigerate for 2 hours. Bring to room temperature 30 minutes before cooking.

Place lamb in a roasting pan, pour half the stock around, cover pan with foil and roast at 160C for 1½ hours, then remove foil, baste with pan juices and roast another 30 minutes or until lamb is browned. Remove lamb from pan and rest in a warm place for 10 minutes. Skim fat from juices in pan, add chicken stock and cook over high heat until reduced by half, then season to taste.

Meanwhile, place vegetables in a large roasting pan, drizzle with a little olive oil, toss to coat and roast at 160C for 1 hour. While lamb is resting, increase heat to 200C and roast vegetables another 10 minutes until golden. Just before serving, toss vegetables with parsley and currants and serve with sliced lamb drizzled with pan juices.

SERVES 4

rack of lamb with quinoa and roasted pumpkin

Ask your butcher to French trim the racks of lamb. This means that he will cut off all the fat and leave you with just meat, and he will also clean the bones, but it's simple enough to do yourself.

½ butternut pumpkin, peeled and cut into 2 cm pieces

olive oil

2 x 6-cutlet racks of lamb, French trimmed

1 onion, chopped

1 baby fennel bulb, trimmed and chopped

2 cloves garlic, chopped

500 ml (2 cups) Chicken Stock (page 159)

190 g (1 cup) quinoa

¼ cup chopped fresh mixed herbs including basil, mint, flat-leaf parsley

½ cup Hummus (page 165)

100 g baby spinach leaves, to serve

Place pumpkin on an oven tray, brush with a little oil and roast at 200°C about 20–30 minutes, turning once, or until pumpkin is golden and tender.

Brush lamb with a little oil and cook in a hot non-stick frying pan until browned. Transfer to an oven tray and roast at 200°C for 15 minutes for pink lamb. Remove from oven, cover loosely with foil and rest in a warm place for 10 minutes before slicing into cutlets.

Meanwhile, heat 1 tablespoon olive oil in a saucepan, add onion, fennel, and garlic and cook over low heat for 5 minutes. Add 60 ml (¼ cup) of the stock and cook, covered, over low heat about 20 minutes or until fennel is soft. Add quinoa and remaining stock, bring to a simmer and cook, covered, about 15 minutes or until quinoa is tender. Remove from heat, season to taste and gently stir in pumpkin and herbs.

Serve Hummus topped with quinoa and pumpkin mixture, baby spinach leaves and sliced lamb cutlets.

SERVES 4

Best made just before serving.

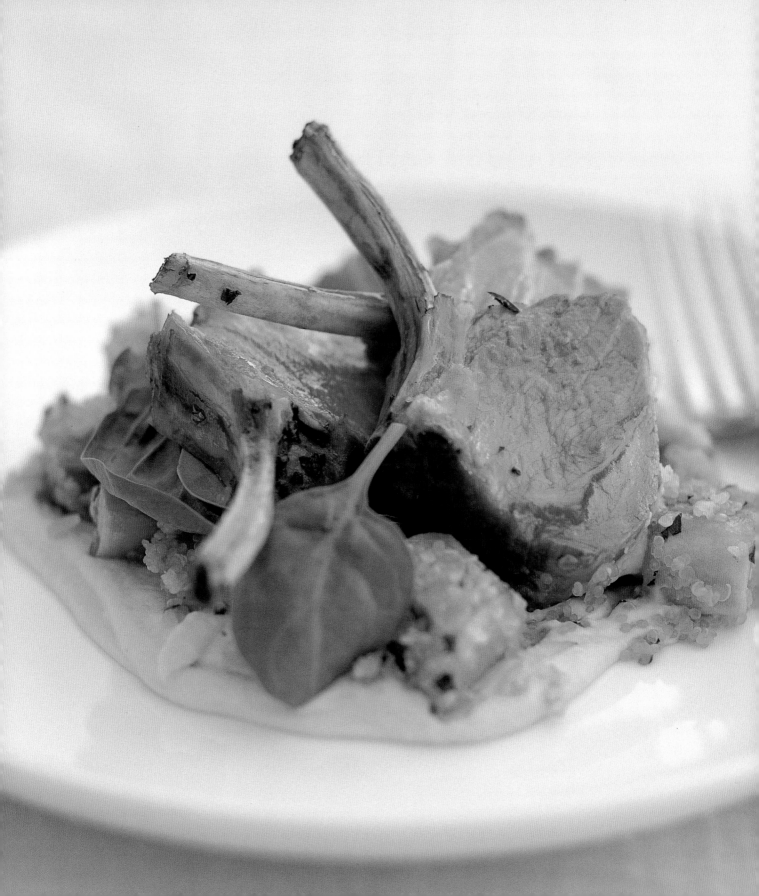

crisp ocean trout with wilted spinach & mushy peas

When you are serving fillets of fish, it is implied that there are no bones, so make sure you remove them. You can buy giant-sized tweezers from kitchen shops that do the trick really well. As well as tasting fabulous, this is a very pretty dish and is suitable to serve for a dinner party.

800 g orange sweet potato, cut into
  2 cm pieces

olive oil

500 ml (2 cups) Chicken Stock
  (page 159)

1 kg peas, podded

2 tsp butter

4 ocean trout fillets (180 g each),
  skinned and pinboned

2 bunches English spinach, trimmed

Place sweet potato on an oven tray, brush with a little oil and roast at 200°C, turning once, about 30 minutes or until browned and tender.

Bring chicken stock to the boil, add peas and cook, uncovered, over medium heat about 8 minutes or until tender. Drain and reserve stock. Refresh peas under cold water. Return peas to pan, add a little reserved stock and butter and mash with a potato masher until coarsely crushed, then season to taste.

Brush skinned side of ocean trout with oil and sprinkle with sea salt. Heat a non-stick frying pan until hot and cook trout over high heat about 2 minutes or until browned. Turn and cook another minute for a pink centre, or until fish is cooked to your liking.

Meanwhile, place spinach in a large saucepan and cook, covered, over medium heat until just wilted. Drain and rinse under cold water, then squeeze out excess. Return to pan, season to taste and toss over heat with a drizzle of olive oil. Spoon wilted spinach onto plates, top with mushy peas and ocean trout and place roasted sweet potato to one side.

SERVES 4

Best made just before serving.

caponata with chargrilled garfish

Small red mullet or sardines can be used for this recipe instead of garfish. Allow 2 red mullet or 3 sardines per person for a main course. All these fish have quite a lot of bones, but you can get around that by asking your fishmonger to butterfly the garfish or the sardines if that worries you.

18 garfish, cleaned

olive oil

100 g baby rocket leaves

lemon wedges, to serve

CAPONATA

500 g eggplant, cut into 2 cm pieces

1 red and 1 yellow capsicum, cut into
 2 cm pieces

olive oil

1 red (Spanish) onion, chopped

2 sticks celery, chopped

2 cloves garlic, chopped

1 x 400 g can tomatoes

2 tbsp red wine vinegar or apple cider
 vinegar

1/4 tsp honey

2 tbsp baby olives, pitted

1 tbsp salt-packed capers, rinsed

1/4 cup fresh flat-leaf parsley leaves

To make Caponata, place eggplant and capsicum on an oven tray, toss with a little oil and roast at 200°C for 20 minutes or until browned on edges.

Heat 1 tablespoon oil in a saucepan and cook onion and celery over low heat until soft, adding a little water if onion is sticking to pan. Add garlic, tomatoes, vinegar and honey, season to taste and cook, uncovered, over medium heat until tomatoes are reduced and pulpy. Stir in eggplant and capsicum, olives and capers and simmer another 5 minutes. Check seasoning and stir in parsley.

Brush garfish lightly with oil and chargrill or barbecue over high heat on both sides until cooked (about 2 minutes each side).

Place a pile of rocket leaves on each plate and top with garfish. Serve caponata and lemon wedges to one side.

SERVES 6

Caponata can be made a day ahead. Add parsley just before serving. Will keep, covered, in refrigerator.

silver bream en papilotte with ginger & eschallots

Cooking in a foil or baking paper package is a simple technique that ensures the fish remains moist and full of flavour. You can try this with fish fillets as well and it works particularly well with salmon. Serve it straight from the parcel if you like.

4 silver bream or baby snapper, about 350 g each

16 sprigs fresh coriander

4 cm piece ginger, shredded

80 ml (1/3 cup) Chicken Stock (page 159)

1 tbsp rice wine vinegar

light olive oil

1/2 (700 g) Chinese white cabbage, finely shredded

2 eschallots, finely sliced

2 tbsp soy sauce or wheat-free tamari sauce

2 tsp sesame oil

4 green (spring) onions, shredded lengthwise

steamed rice, cooked according to directions on packet, to serve

Pat fish dry with absorbent paper, then place each in the centre of a large piece of foil or baking paper. Place half the coriander and ginger in cavities of fish and top with the rest, then drizzle with stock and rice wine vinegar. Fold foil over to form parcels, then place on 2 oven trays and roast at 200°C for 10–15 minutes depending on thickness of fish. Remove from oven and stand for 5 minutes before serving.

Meanwhile, heat a little oil in a wok and stir-fry cabbage and eschallots until just wilted, then season to taste.

Open parcels and transfer fish to plates with their juices. Drizzle with soy sauce and sesame oil and sprinkle with green onions. Serve with stir-fried cabbage and eschallots and steamed rice.

SERVES 4

Best made just before serving.

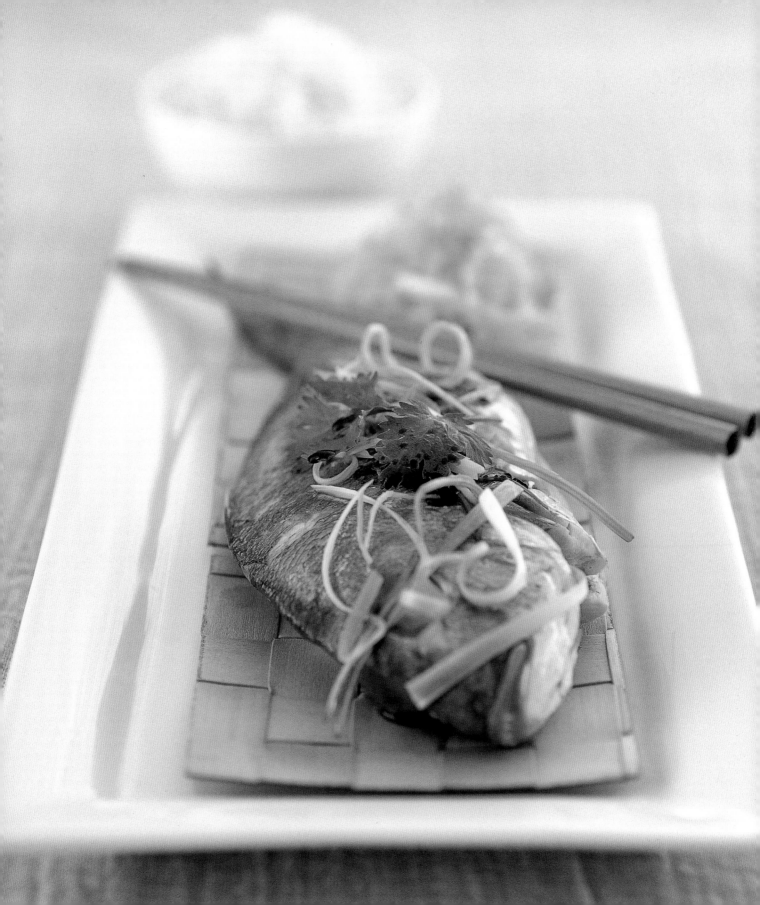

baked snapper with braised fennel & leeks and lentils

As an alternative technique, the snapper for this dish can be baked in a salt crust. You will need 1 kg sea salt (available from supermarkets). Line a large baking tray with foil and sprinkle with one third of the salt. Place unscaled fish on top of salt and fill cavity with 1 sliced lemon and 4 sprigs of thyme. Place remaining salt over fish to cover, leaving head and tail exposed. Bring foil up around fish to contain the salt on the sides. Roast at 200°C for 30 minutes. Remove from oven and stand 15 minutes before removing crust. Gently peel away skin and serve with braised leeks and fennel.

4 leeks, trimmed and halved lengthwise

1 large fennel bulb, trimmed, cored and
   sliced into wedges

8 sprigs fresh thyme

300 ml Chicken Stock (page 159)

2 kg whole snapper, gutted and scaled

extra virgin olive oil

1 lemon, sliced

200 g (1 cup) French green (Puy) lentils

2 vine-ripened tomatoes, peeled,
   seeded and chopped

extra fresh thyme sprigs, to serve

lemon juice, to serve

Place leeks, fennel and half the thyme sprigs in a large roasting pan. Pour stock over vegetables, then cover with foil and roast at 200°C for 30 minutes. Remove from oven and remove foil.

Brush snapper lightly with oil and place remaining thyme with lemon slices in cavity. Place snapper over vegetables and season to taste. Return to oven and roast, uncovered, about 30 minutes or until dorsal fin (along the back bone) can be removed easily.

Remove snapper to a plate, cover loosely with foil and rest in a warm place for 10 minutes. Keep vegetables warm.

Meanwhile, cook lentils, uncovered, in simmering water about 20 minutes or until tender. Drain. Return lentils to pan, add tomato and season to taste.

Using a fork and spoon, remove skin from fish. Remove fish from bones.

Spoon lentil mixture onto plates, top with fennel and leek mixture and snapper. Sprinkle with extra thyme. Drizzle with a little oil and lemon juice.

SERVES 6

Best made just before serving.

seared barramundi with braised chickpeas & herb yoghurt

You could make this dish with salmon or snapper. The Braised Chickpeas are also an excellent base for a simple soup with wilted spinach stirred through. The added bonus is that everything can be prepared in advance and all you have to do is cook the fish at the last minute.

olive oil

6 x 200 g fillets wild barramundi, skinned

400 g baby beans, trimmed and blanched, to serve

BRAISED CHICKPEAS

100 g (1/2 cup) dried chickpeas, soaked in cold water overnight

olive oil

1 red (Spanish) onion, sliced

750 ml (3 cups) Chicken Stock (page 159)

4 vine-ripened tomatoes, peeled, seeded and coarsely chopped

2 cloves garlic, chopped

good pinch saffron threads, to taste

HERB YOGHURT

1 cup plain soy yoghurt

1 clove garlic, crushed

2 tbsp lemon juice

1/4 cup mixed fresh herbs, including basil, flat-leaf parsley and coriander, chopped

To make Herb Yoghurt, combine all ingredients and season to taste.

To make Braised Chickpeas, cook chickpeas, uncovered, in simmering water about 30 minutes or until tender. Drain.

Heat 1 tablespoon oil in a large frying pan and cook onion over low heat until soft, adding a little stock if onion is sticking to pan. Add half the stock, tomatoes and garlic and cook, uncovered, over high heat until tomatoes are thick and pulpy. Add remaining stock, saffron and chickpeas and simmer another 10 minutes, then season to taste.

Heat a little oil in a non-stick frying pan and cook barramundi, skinned side first, over medium heat about 2 minutes or until golden, turn and cook another 2 minutes or until fish is just cooked.

Divide chickpea mixture among shallow bowls, top with blanched beans and barramundi and drizzle with Herb Yoghurt.

SERVES 6

Chickpea and tomato mixture can be made 3 hours ahead. Will keep, covered, at room temperature.

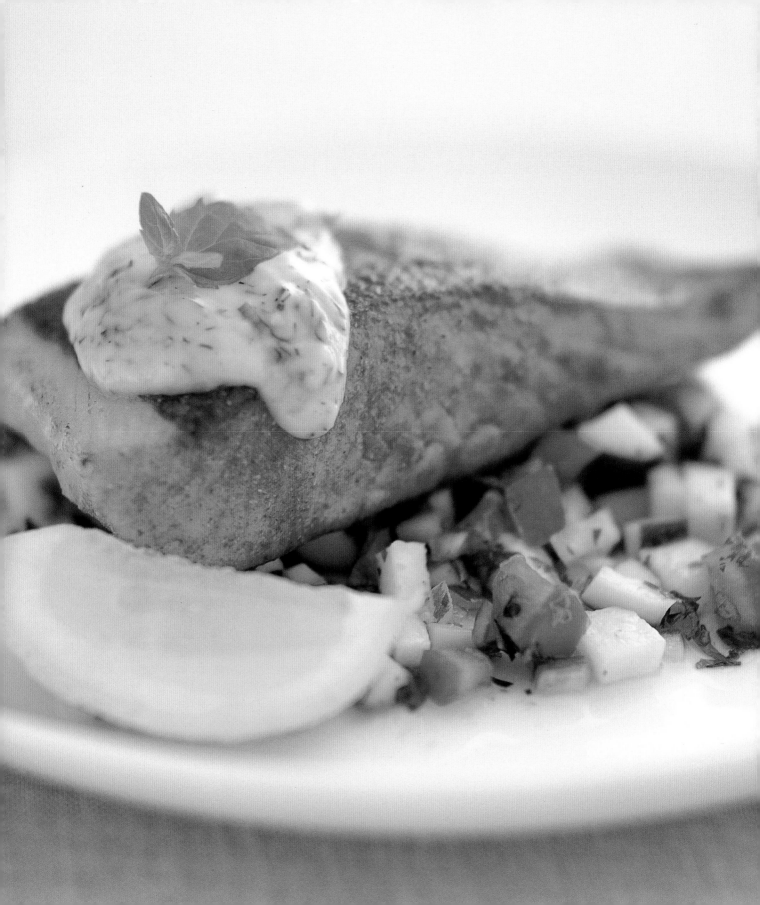

spice-crusted ocean trout with zucchini salad

Check that you are using sweet paprika in the spice crust for this dish — hot paprika would overpower the flavour of the fish. You could also serve the fish on a bed of wilted spinach with some roasted vegetables, such as eggplant and capsicum.

2 tsp ground coriander

2 tsp ground cumin

1 tsp ground sweet paprika

1 tsp fine sea salt

4 x 180 g ocean trout fillets

1 tbsp olive oil

$\frac{1}{2}$ cup Yoghurt Dressing (page 164), to serve

Leafy Green Salad (page 161) and lemon wedges, to serve

ZUCCHINI SALAD

2 zucchini, chopped into 1 cm pieces

$\frac{1}{2}$ red (Spanish) onion, finely chopped

2 vine-ripened tomatoes, seeded and chopped into 1 cm pieces

1 Lebanese (small green) cucumber, peeled, seeded and chopped into 1 cm pieces

2 tbsp chopped fresh mint

2 tbsp chopped fresh flat-leaf parsley

1 tbsp olive oil

1 tbsp lemon juice

To make Zucchini Salad, combine all ingredients and season to taste.

Combine coriander, cumin, paprika and salt and rub over fish. Stand for 30 minutes for flavours to develop.

Heat oil in a non-stick frying pan and cook fish about 2 minutes each side or until cooked to your liking.

Serve Zucchini Salad topped with fish and a drizzle of Yoghurt Dressing, with lemon wedges and Leafy Green Salad.

SERVES 4

Zucchini Salad can be made 3 hours ahead.
Will keep, covered, at room temperature.

whiting with tomato & saffron broth & zucchini ribbons

Whiting has a beautiful delicate flavour and lends itself well to steaming, which is such a gentle form of cooking. With no other added flavours, you get the real benefit of the taste of the fish. You could use another white fish like snapper or bream if you can't get whiting.

4 vine-ripened tomatoes, peeled,
    seeded and chopped
750 ml Fish or Chicken Stock
    (pages 159 & 160)
¼ tsp saffron threads, soaked in 1 tbsp
    hot water for 10 minutes
1 dried bay leaf
4 zucchini, cut lengthwise into ribbons
12 x 50 g fillets of whiting, skinned
400 g chat potatoes
extra virgin olive oil
2 tsp fresh thyme leaves, plus a few
    sprigs of fresh thyme

Combine tomatoes, stock and saffron mixture and puree in a food processor in 2 batches until smooth. Place mixture in a saucepan, add bay leaf, bring to the boil and simmer, uncovered, for 10 minutes, then season to taste. Remove bay leaf.

Place zucchini ribbons in the top of a steamer over simmering water, cover and steam about 4 minutes or until just tender. Remove from steamer and keep warm.

Line steamer with baking paper and add half the whiting. Cover and steam about 2 minutes or until just cooked. Remove and keep warm. Repeat with remaining whiting.

Meanwhile cook potatoes, uncovered, in simmering salted water until tender. Drain, halve lengthwise, toss with a little olive oil and thyme leaves and season to taste.

Place zucchini ribbons in the base of shallow bowls, pour tomato broth around and top with steamed whiting, a drizzle of oil and a few sprigs of thyme. Serve with potatoes.

SERVES 4

Tomato & Saffron Broth can be made 3 hours ahead.
Will keep, covered, at room temperature.

fish stew with white beans & roasted garlic toasts

This lovely stew is ideal to serve at a party and also doubles well as an entree for about 10 people. Roast the spices in a dry non-stick pan until aromatic – this will intensify their flavour and remove the 'raw' taste.

200 g (1 cup) dried cannellini beans, soaked overnight in cold water

2 knobs (heads) garlic

olive oil

2 leeks, chopped

1 tsp fennel seeds, roasted and coarsely ground

1 tsp cumin seeds, roasted and coarsely ground

2 cloves garlic, chopped

6 vine-ripened tomatoes, peeled, seeded and chopped

400 g desiree potatoes, chopped

2 dried bay leaves

1.5 L (6 cups) Fish or Chicken Stock (pages 159 & 160)

500 g black mussels, scrubbed and bearded

12 medium green prawns, peeled and deveined

3 medium calamari, cleaned and cut into strips

400 g firm white fish, cut into 3 cm pieces

1/3 cup shredded fresh coriander

rye or gluten-free bread, toasted, to serve

Cook cannellini beans, uncovered, in simmering water about 30 minutes or until tender. Drain.

Wrap garlic in foil and roast on an oven tray at 200°C about 30 minutes or until cloves are tender. When cool enough to handle, squeeze garlic from cloves and place in a small bowl, then mash until smooth.

Heat 1 tablespoon oil in a large heavy-based saucepan and cook leek, covered, over low heat until soft. Add ground fennel and cumin and cook about 1 minute until aromatic. Add extra chopped garlic and tomatoes and cook, uncovered, over high heat until tomatoes are pulpy. Add potatoes, bay leaves and stock, season to taste and simmer over medium heat until potatoes are just cooked, then add drained beans and simmer another 5 minutes. Add mussels and cook, covered, over medium heat until mussels have opened. Add remaining seafood, cover and cook over low heat about 5 minutes or until seafood is just cooked. Stir in coriander.

Serve in shallow bowls with toasted bread spread with mashed garlic.

SERVES 6

Recipe can be prepared 3 hours ahead. Add seafood just before serving. Will keep, covered, at room temperature.

barbecued seafood with mango salsa & pink potato salad

This is the perfect dish for entertaining in the summer and is ideal for serving outdoors. It's simple, most of the cooking is last minute and you can vary the seafood you use depending on what is fresh and looks good on the day.

Mixed seafood to barbecue, including
  small fish and shellfish such as
  garfish or red mullet, prawns, baby
  squid hoods or butterflied sardines
olive oil
rocket leaves and lemon wedges,
  to serve

PINK POTATO SALAD

1 egg yolk

1 tbsp lemon juice

1/2 tsp Dijon mustard

1 clove garlic

75 ml olive oil

1/4 Roasted Capsicum (page 163),
  chopped

1 kg baby chat potatoes

MANGO SALSA

1 mango, finely chopped

1/2 small red (Spanish) onion, finely
  chopped

1/2 avocado, seeded, peeled and finely
  chopped

2 tbsp lemon juice

1 tbsp chopped fresh mint

To make Pink Potato Salad, combine egg yolk, lemon juice, mustard and garlic in a bowl with a small hand-held blender and blend until smooth. With motor operating, add oil in a thin stream until thick, then add 1 tablespoon water and blend until smooth. Add capsicum, season to taste and blend until smooth. Cook potatoes, uncovered, in simmering salted water until tender. Drain and cool. Toss potatoes in pink mayonnaise.

To make Mango Salsa, combine all ingredients and season to taste.

Brush fish and seafood with olive oil and barbecue or chargrill until cooked.

Serve fish and lemon wedges on a large platter on a bed of rocket with Pink Potato Salad and Mango Salsa served separately.

SERVES 6–8

Pink Potato Salad and Mango Salsa can be prepared 3 hours ahead. Toss potatoes with pink mayonnaise just before serving. Mayonnaise and salsa will keep, covered, in refrigerator, and potatoes will keep at room temperature.

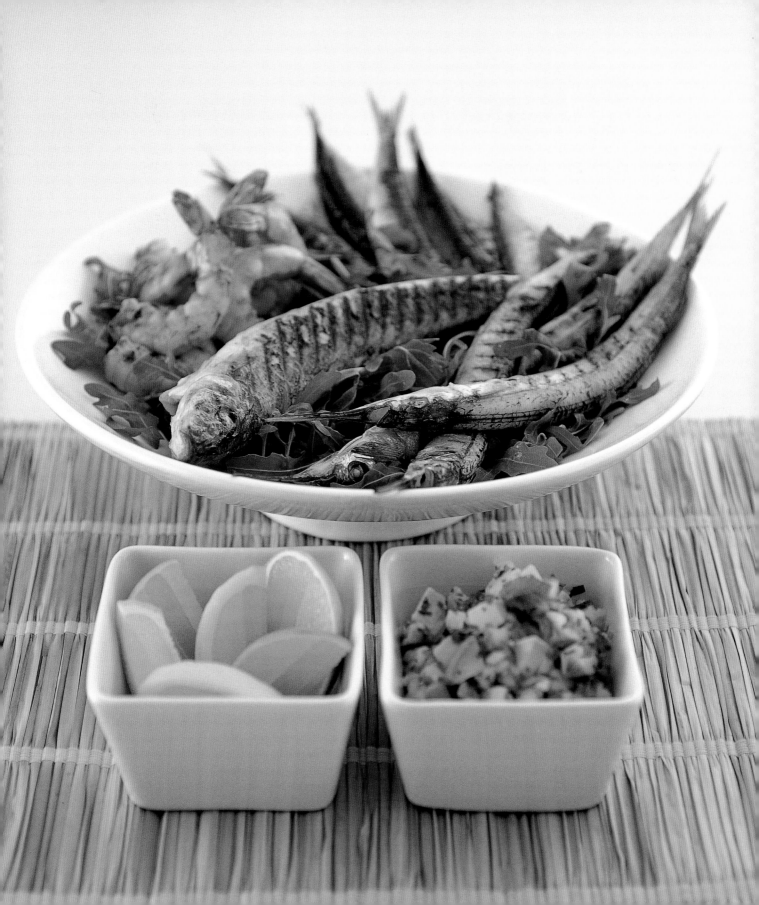

poached salmon with nicoise salad

You can never have too much poached salmon! It's a wonderful dish served whole for a large gathering, or for a smaller group you can simply poach individual fillets in a pan of water with the flavourings used below. Bring the court bouillon (the poaching liquid) to the boil with the salmon fillets in the pan. As soon as the water starts to bubble, remove from heat and stand salmon about 7 minutes, depending on thickness of fillet.

2.5 kg whole salmon, cleaned and
  scaled

1 small onion, sliced

2 dried bay leaves

6 sprigs fresh parsley

6 black peppercorns

250 ml (1 cup) Light Mayonnaise
  (page 164)

2 tbsp chopped fresh dill

NICOISE SALAD

2 punnets cherry tomatoes, halved

500 g baby beans, trimmed and
  blanched

1 kg kipfler or other waxy potatoes,
  boiled until tender, peeled and sliced

90 g (1/2 cup) baby olives, pitted

1 tbsp olive oil

2 tbsp lemon juice

Remove salmon from refrigerator and bring to room temperature. Wipe fish inside and out with absorbent paper making sure any blood is removed from inside the fish as this can result in a bitter taste. Place fish on rack in a fish kettle, cover with cold water, add onion, bay leaves, parsley and peppercorns. Cover fish kettle with a lid, place over two burners on the cook top and bring slowly to the boil (this will take about 15 minutes). As soon as water begins to bubble, turn off heat and remove lid, to begin the cooling process.

Leave fish to cool in poaching liquid so that it remains very moist and retains all its flavour. The salmon is cooked when dorsal fin (the large one along the backbone) comes out easily when pulled. A 2.5 kg fish will take 1½–2 hours to finish cooking once heat has been turned off.

Remove fish from poaching liquid, place on a serving plate and remove skin and surface bones. Skin will come away quite easily in large sheets. Gently scrape away any dark flesh on the surface of the fish and leave head and tail intact if you intend to serve it whole.

Meanwhile, to make Nicoise Salad, combine all ingredients in a large bowl, season to taste and toss gently. Spoon salad onto plates, top with portions of salmon and drizzle with combined Light Mayonnaise and dill.

SERVES 10–12

Nicoise Salad can be made 3 hours ahead.
Will keep, covered, at room temperature.

chargrilled tuna with kipfler potatoes

We love this dish for its simplicity. If you can't get kipfler potatoes, use some other waxy potato that will stay firm. About ten years ago, there were only two types of potato – washed and unwashed. Today we have a greater choice, so it's best to look for the most suitable potato.

600 g kipfler potatoes

4 x 200 g tuna steaks

olive oil

2 bunches broccolini, trimmed and
   blanched, to serve

lemon wedges, to serve

GREEN OLIVE SALSA

80 g (^{1}/2 cup) green olives, pitted and
   finely chopped

1 small red (Spanish) onion, finely
   chopped

1 tbsp salt-packed capers, rinsed

1 cup firmly packed fresh flat-leaf
   parsley leaves

1 tbsp lemon juice

1 tbsp olive oil

To make Green Olive Salsa, combine all ingredients and season to taste.

Cook potatoes, uncovered, in simmering salted water until tender, then drain. When cool enough to handle, peel and cut into 1 cm thick rounds.

Toss Green Olive Salsa with potatoes.

Brush tuna lightly with olive oil and chargrill about 2 minutes each side for a rare centre or until cooked to your liking.

Serve potato mixture topped with tuna and place broccolini and lemon wedges to one side.

SERVES 4

Green Olive Salsa can be made 3 hours ahead.
Will keep, covered, at room temperature.

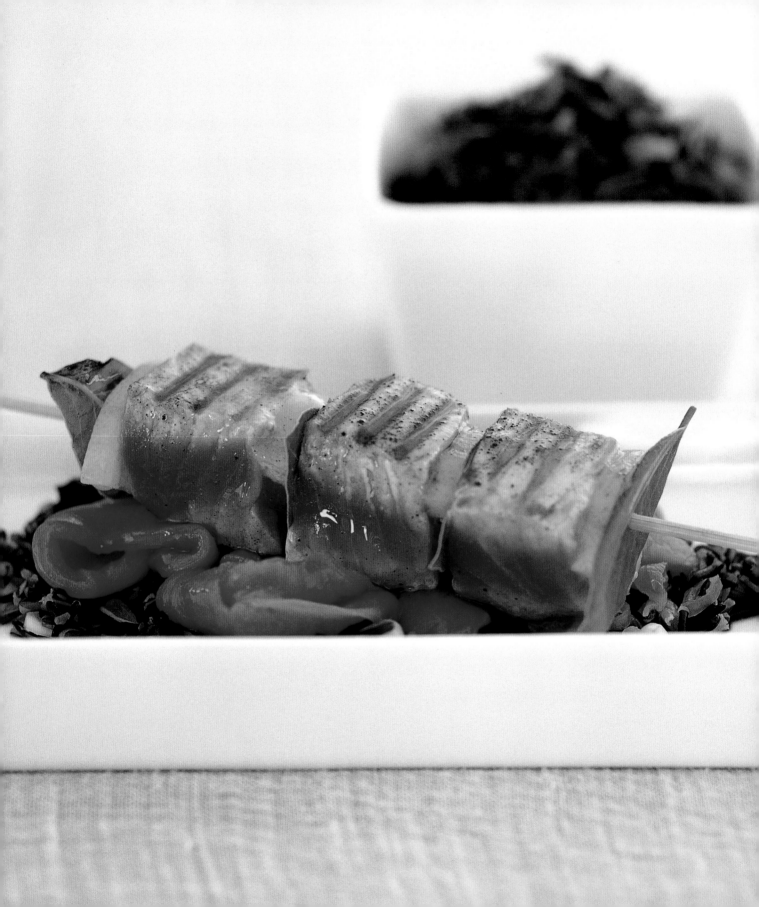

tuna & bay leaf kebabs with wild rice & spinach salad

In the past we have made this recipe using swordfish. However, because of recent concerns over the mercury levels in swordfish, we have switched to tuna. You could also use Spanish mackerel or ocean trout. The fresh bay leaves and lemon wedges add a gorgeous delicate flavour to the fish without overpowering it. The salad is also excellent served with grilled organic lamb or chicken.

1 lemon

24 (approximately) fresh bay leaves

4 bamboo skewers, soaked in cold
  water 30 minutes

1 x 700 g piece tuna, cut into
  3 cm pieces

olive oil

2 Roasted Capsicum (page 163)

WILD RICE & SPINACH SALAD

180 g (1 cup) wild rice

1 bunch English spinach, trimmed

4 green (spring) onions, finely chopped

1/4 preserved lemon, flesh discarded,
  peel rinsed and chopped

1 tbsp lemon juice

1 tbsp extra virgin olive oil

To make Wild Rice & Spinach Salad, cook wild rice, uncovered, in simmering water about 25 minutes or until tender, then drain and rinse under cold water. Cook washed spinach, covered, in a saucepan over medium heat until just wilted. Drain, rinse under cold water, then squeeze out excess water. Chop spinach, then stir into rice with remaining ingredients and season to taste.

Slice lemon and cut each slice into 4. Place a bay leaf and a quarter slice of lemon on a skewer, followed by a piece of tuna, then repeat several times, finishing with a slice of lemon and a bay leaf. Repeat with remaining skewers, then brush with olive oil.

Chargrill or grill kebabs over medium heat about 2 minutes each side, which will leave them still a little rare in the centre, or cook to your liking.

Serve kebabs on a bed of Wild Rice & Spinach Salad and Roasted Capsicum.

SERVES 4

Wild Rice & Spinach Salad can be made and kebabs can be assembled 3 hours ahead. Salad will keep, covered, at room temperature, and the kebabs will keep, covered, in refrigerator.

grilled rainbow trout with broad bean puree

Celeriac is a wonderful winter vegetable and is suitable for mashing and roasting as well as eating raw. When you peel and slice it and don't intend to use it immediately, you need to put it in some water with lemon juice otherwise it will discolour. If you can't get red witlof, use the regular ones with the green tips. They taste much the same, but it's nice to use the red ones in this salad for the colour.

1.2 kg broad beans, podded

1 clove garlic, chopped

60 ml (¼ cup) lemon juice

1 lemon, sliced

4 sprigs fresh dill

4 x 300 g rainbow trout, cleaned

olive oil

lemon wedges, to serve

CELERIAC & WITLOF SALAD

300 g celeriac, peeled and cut into
  matchsticks

2 red witlof, trimmed, cored and cut
  into julienne

100 g snowpea sprouts, trimmed

60 ml (¼ cup) Light Mayonnaise
  (page 164)

1 tbsp chopped fresh dill

Cook podded broad beans, uncovered, in simmering salted water about 3 minutes or until just tender. Drain, rinse under cold water and peel away skins. Place broad beans in a food processor, add garlic and lemon juice and process, adding enough water to form a smooth puree, then season to taste. Return to pan and reheat gently.

To make Celeriac & Witlof Salad, combine all ingredients and season.

Place sliced lemon and dill sprigs in trout cavities, place on a grill tray and brush with a little oil and season to taste. Grill under medium heat about 5 minutes each side depending on thickness, until cooked to your liking.

Serve fish on warm broad bean puree with Celeriac & Witlof Salad and lemon wedges to one side.

SERVES 4

Celeriac & Witlof Salad and broad bean puree can be made 3 hours ahead. Will keep, covered, at room temperature.

braised calamari with lemon & oregano potatoes

Calamari are a bit tricky to cook. You have to cook them really quickly or long and slowly, otherwise it will be tough and chewy. Here we braised stuffed calamari over low heat for an hour so they melt in your mouth. You could serve the calamari and braising liquid with steamed rice as an alternative to the lemon and oregano potatoes. Ask your fishmonger to clean the calamari, but make sure they are fresh. If you are sensitive to shellfish, substitute finely chopped white fish for the prawns.

12 medium green prawns, peeled,
   deveined and finely chopped

1/2 cup finely chopped fresh flat-leaf
   parsley

1 tbsp grated lemon rind

4 x 250 g calamari, cleaned

1 tbsp olive oil

1 onion, chopped

500 ml Chicken Stock (page 159)

2 cloves garlic, chopped

1 x 400 g can tomatoes

Leafy Green Salad (page 161), to serve

LEMON & OREGANO POTATOES

800 g King Edward or desiree potatoes,
   peeled and chopped into 4 cm pieces

2 lemons, chopped into 4 cm pieces

1 knob (head) garlic, cloves separated

2 tbsp olive oil

1/3 cup fresh oregano leaves

Combine prawns, parsley and lemon rind and season to taste. Spoon mixture into calamari hoods and secure openings with a toothpick.

Heat oil in a deep frying pan and cook onion over low heat until soft, adding a little stock if onion is sticking to pan. Add garlic, tomatoes and stock and cook, uncovered, over high heat until reduced by half, then season to taste. Add calamari, cover partially with a lid and cook over low heat, turning occasionally, about 1 hour or until calamari are tender.

Meanwhile, to make Lemon & Oregano Potatoes, place potatoes and lemon in a roasting pan, toss with oil and roast at 200°C for 30 minutes, turning occasionally. Add garlic and cook another 30 minutes until potatoes and lemons are browned and garlic is soft. Remove from oven and stir in oregano.

Serve calamari and braising sauce with Lemon & Oregano Potatoes and Leafy Green Salad.

SERVES 4

Calamari can be braised 2 hours ahead and reheated gently. Will keep, covered, at room temperature.

eggplant stack with sweet potato mash & salsa verde

We are quite conservative in our suggestions for how far ahead you can prepare various dishes. The salsa verde here could be prepared a day ahead, however we feel it loses its freshness and the herbs lose their colour. As most of these dishes are simple to prepare, our preference is to cook and serve on the day.

500 g orange sweet potato, peeled and chopped

1 clove garlic, chopped

1 tsp ground cumin

1 tsp ground coriander

1 tbsp lemon juice

olive oil

500 g eggplant, sliced crosswise into 1 cm thick slices (8 slices)

2 zucchini, sliced 1 cm thick on diagonal

250 g firm tofu, sliced into 1 cm thick slices

1 Roasted Capsicum (page 163)

100 g snowpea sprouts

SALSA VERDE

1 cup firmly packed mixed fresh herbs, including basil, coriander, dill and mint

1 clove garlic, chopped

1 tsp Dijon mustard

1 tsp capers, drained

1 tbsp lemon juice

1 tbsp olive oil

To make Salsa Verde, combine all ingredients in a food processor and process until smooth, then season to taste.

Cook sweet potato in simmering salted water, uncovered, over medium heat about 10 minutes or until tender, then drain. Place sweet potato in a food processor with garlic, ground spices, lemon juice and 1 tablespoon oil and process until smooth, then season to taste.

Place eggplant and zucchini on an oven tray, toss with 1 tablespoon oil and roast at 200°C for 30 minutes, turning once, until browned and tender.

Pat tofu dry with absorbent paper, brush with a little oil and chargrill or grill on both sides until lightly browned.

Spoon sweet potato mash onto plates and top with layered vegetables, capsicum and tofu and a spoonful of Salsa Verde. Serve snowpea sprouts to one side.

SERVES 4

Salsa Verde can be made 3 hours ahead.
Will keep, covered, at room temperature.

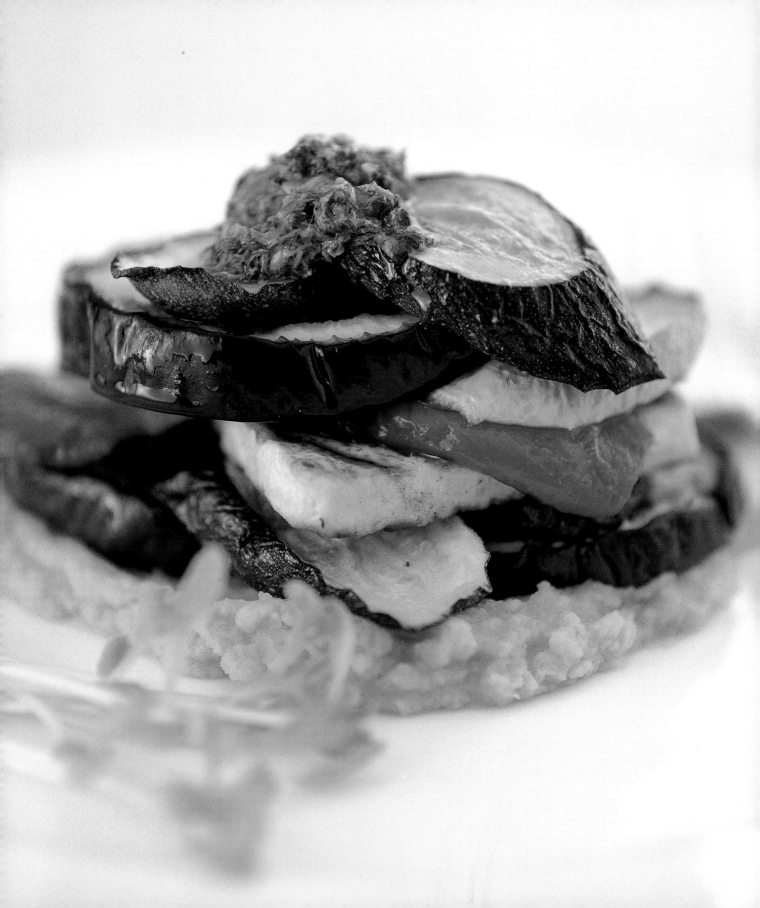

beetroot & buckwheat risotto with crushed pinenuts

Vegetarians and non-vegetarians alike will enjoy this dish. The addition of buckwheat to the risotto gives it more body and chew. It's also lovely served with some sliced roasted venison or lamb, or roasted quail.

4 beetroot, trimmed

olive oil

1 onion, chopped

2 cloves garlic, chopped

200 g (1 cup) arborio rice

200 g (1 cup) whole raw buckwheat

1 L (4 cups) Vegetable or Chicken Stock (page 159), approximately

2 tsp butter

2 tbsp chopped fresh chives

2 tbsp pinenuts, toasted and coarsely crushed with a mortar and pestle

Wrap beetroot in foil, then place on an oven tray and roast at 200°C about 50–60 minutes or until tender. Remove foil and, when cool enough to handle, peel away skins. Cut beetroot into 1 cm pieces.

Heat 1 tablespoon oil in a saucepan, add onion and cook over low heat until soft. Add garlic, rice and buckwheat and stir to coat in oil and toast lightly. Have stock simmering in another saucepan.

Add 250 ml (1 cup) stock to rice mixture and stir over low to medium heat until stock is absorbed. Add remaining stock 125 ml ($\frac{1}{2}$ cup) at a time stirring continuously, allowing each addition to be absorbed before adding the next, until rice is just tender (al dente). Stir in beetroot, butter and half the chives with the last addition of stock. Remove from heat and cover with a lid for 5 minutes. Stir in pinenuts and serve in shallow bowls topped with remaining chives.

SERVES 4

Recipe best made just before serving. Beetroot can be roasted a day ahead. Will keep, covered, in refrigerator.

mushroom & eggplant ragout with black eye beans

You could use a variety of dried beans in this dish – try making it with borlotti beans or red kidney beans. Remember not to salt the water when cooking dried beans, as it will make them tough.

100 g (½ cup) dried black eye beans,
  soaked in cold water overnight

1 eggplant (about 400 g), chopped into
  3 cm pieces

1 red capsicum, chopped into 3 cm
  pieces

olive oil

1 large onion, chopped

1 tsp ground coriander

1 tsp ground cumin

400 g Swiss brown or small cap
  mushrooms, stalks trimmed

60 ml (¼ cup) Vegetable Stock
  (page 159) or water

3 cloves garlic, chopped

1 tbsp lemon juice

55 g (⅓ cup) raisins

2 tbsp chopped fresh mint

2 tbsp chopped fresh flat-leaf parsley

basmati rice, steamed according to
  directions on packet, to serve

Cook drained beans in simmering water, uncovered, about 30 minutes or until beans are tender. Drain.

Place eggplant and capsicum on an oven tray, toss with 1 tablespoon oil and roast at 200°C about 20 minutes, turning once, or until tender and golden.

Heat 1 tablespoon oil in a large saucepan and cook onion and spices over low heat until onion is soft and spices are aromatic, adding a little water if onion is sticking to pan. Increase heat, add mushrooms and cook until lightly browned. Add stock or water, beans, garlic, lemon juice, raisins, eggplant and capsicum, season to taste and cook, covered, over low heat 15 minutes. Stir in mint and parsley and serve with steamed rice.

SERVES 4

Ragout can be made a day ahead and reheated gently.
Will keep, covered, in refrigerator.

hot & spicy vegetable tagine with chickpeas

There is a bit of chopping to do, but once the preparation is done it is a very simple dish to bring together and you will be rewarded by the result. The Spice Mix also works well with chicken and it can be made ahead of time and stored in an airtight container.

100 g (½ cup) dried chickpeas, soaked in cold water overnight

2 tbsp olive oil

1 large onion, thinly sliced

1 large fresh red chilli, seeded and chopped

1 red capsicum, chopped

4 cloves garlic, chopped

2 carrots, chopped

300 g orange sweet potato, peeled and chopped

4 vine-ripened tomatoes, chopped

300 g desiree potatoes, peeled and chopped

1 stick celery, sliced

200 g green beans, trimmed, halved

Yoghurt Dressing (page 164), to serve

SPICE MIX

1 tbsp cumin seeds, roasted

1 tbsp coriander seeds, roasted

2 tsp sweet paprika

1 tsp sea salt

½ tsp cayenne pepper

½ tsp finely ground black pepper

Cook drained chickpeas in simmering water, uncovered, about 30 minutes or until tender. Drain.

To make Spice Mix, combine all spices and grind in a spice grinder or small food processor until fine.

Heat oil in a large heavy-based casserole and cook onion, chilli, capsicum and 2 tablespoons of the spice mix over low heat until onion is soft, adding a little water if onion is sticking to pan. Reserve any remaining spice mix for another use.

Add chickpeas, garlic, remaining vegetables and 250 ml (1 cup) water and season to taste. Cook, covered, over low heat about 30 minutes or until vegetables are tender. Serve drizzled with Yoghurt Dressing.

SERVES 4–6

Recipe can be made a day ahead and reheated gently.
Will keep, covered, in refrigerator.

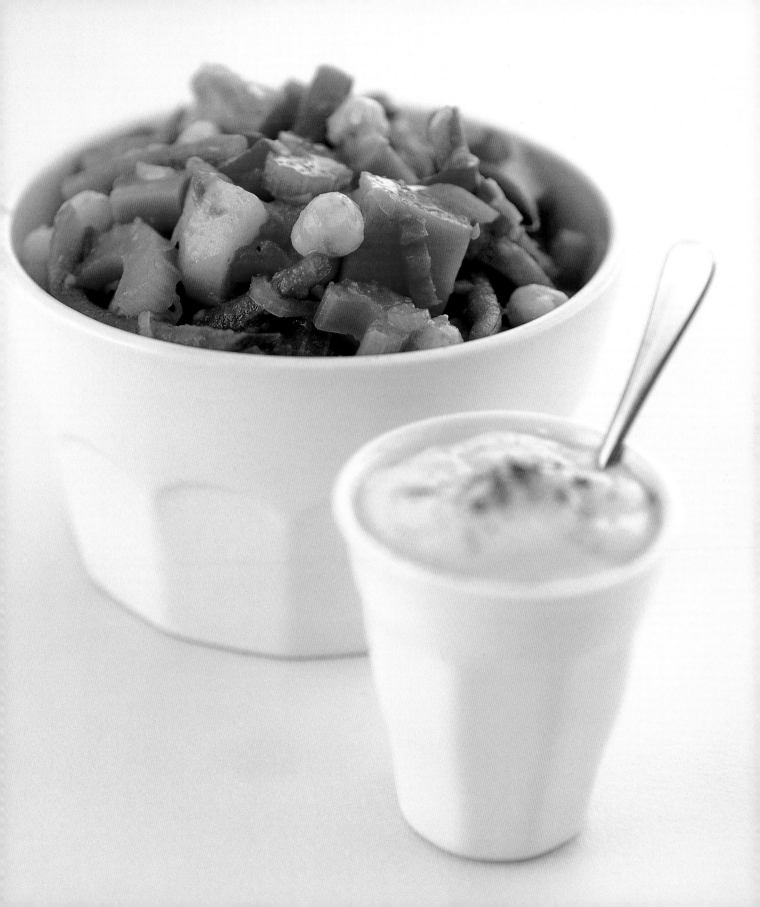

spinach gnocchi with tomatoes & pinenuts

It is important when making gnocchi to add just enough flour to bring the potato mixture together to form a smooth dough, otherwise they will be tough and chewy. You can also serve the gnocchi with our Tomato, Red Lentil & Black Olive Sauce (page 77).

1 bunch English spinach, trimmed

900 g sebago potatoes, peeled and chopped

1 egg, lightly whisked

115 g ($^3/_4$ cup) all-purpose gluten-free flour mix, approximately

extra virgin olive oil

4 vine-ripened tomatoes, coarsely chopped

2 cloves garlic, chopped

2 tbsp pinenuts, toasted

freshly ground black pepper

2 tbsp fresh baby basil leaves

Leafy Green Salad (page 161), to serve

Cook spinach, covered, in a large saucepan over low heat until just wilted. Drain and rinse under cold water, then squeeze out excess moisture. Cool and chop finely.

Cook potatoes, uncovered, in simmering salted water until just tender. Drain and, when cool enough to handle, push through a ricer or a mouli. Place potato in a bowl, season to taste and stir in spinach and egg.

Place potato mixture on work surface, sprinkle with flour 37 g ($^1/_4$ cup) at a time and knead to form a smooth dough. You might need to add a bit less or more flour depending on wetness of potato. Divide potato mixture into four and roll each piece of dough into a log. Using a sharp knife, cut log into 2 cm pieces.

Bring a large saucepan of water to the boil, reduce heat, add salt and cook gnocchi in batches until they rise to the surface. Remove with a slotted spoon and place in bowls.

Meanwhile, heat 1 tablespoon oil in a frying pan until hot, add tomatoes and garlic, season to taste and cook over high heat for 2 minutes.

Serve gnocchi topped with tomato mixture, pinenuts, cracked black pepper and basil and a drizzle of oil. Serve with Leafy Green Salad.

SERVES 4

Recipe best made just before serving.

white bean & mushroom 'ravioli' with asparagus & peas

These little parcels are delicious and can be filled with a variety of purees. You could use our Mushroom Pâté (page 91) or the Fennel, Roasted Garlic & White Bean Puree (page 89). It is important that you serve this dish immediately, as the hot stock mixture is what heats the parcels through.

100 g (^{1}/2 cup) dried cannellini beans, soaked in cold water overnight

1 tbsp olive oil

250 g large flat mushrooms, chopped

1 L (4 cups) Vegetable or Chicken Stock (page 159)

2 cloves garlic, chopped

2 tbsp lemon juice

500 g peas, podded

12 spears asparagus, trimmed and halved crosswise

8 x 20 cm rice paper rounds

fresh chives, cut into 4 cm lengths, to serve

Cook drained cannellini beans, uncovered, in simmering water about 30 minutes or until tender. Drain.

Heat oil in a frying pan, add mushrooms and 60 ml (^{1}/4 cup) stock or water and cook over high heat, stirring occasionally, until mushrooms wilt. Add garlic and cook until liquid is evaporated. Combine mushroom mixture, beans and lemon juice in a food processor and process until smooth, then season to taste. Cool slightly.

Bring stock to the boil, add peas and simmer, uncovered, over medium heat about 8 minutes or until peas are tender, then add asparagus and simmer another 2 minutes. Season to taste.

Soak rice paper in hot water, in batches until softened, then place on damp tea towels, covering with another damp tea towel as you work. Spoon 2 tablespoons of pureed mixture into the centre of 1 round and fold in half, pressing edges together to seal. Repeat with remaining rounds and mixture. Place two half rounds in shallow bowls and ladle hot stock mixture over. Sprinkle with chives and serve immediately.

SERVES 4

Recipe best made just before serving.

tofu & vegetable frittata with braised onions

This delicious frittata is very versatile. It's great to take on picnics or you can cut it into small squares and serve it topped with braised onions as an appetiser. Any leftovers can be packed and taken to work for lunch and it can even be eaten as a breakfast dish with roasted tomatoes and mushrooms. Taste the frittata mixture before you bake it to make sure it is well seasoned.

300 g zucchini, coarsely grated

250 g green beans, trimmed

1 bunch English spinach, stalks trimmed, and shredded

200 g firm tofu, drained and coarsely chopped

1 cup chopped fresh mixed herbs including flat-leaf parsley, dill, mint and basil

6 eggs, lightly whisked

50 g (1/3 cup) sesame seeds

Leafy Green Salad (page 161), to serve

BRAISED ONIONS

1 tbsp olive oil

3 red (Spanish) onions, each cut into 8 wedges

60 ml (1/4 cup) Vegetable Stock (page 159) or water

2 tsp fresh thyme leaves

1 tbsp balsamic vinegar

1/4 tsp honey

To make Braised Onions, heat oil in a heavy-based saucepan, add onions and stir over medium heat for 1 minute. Add stock or water, season to taste and cook, covered, over low heat about 30 minutes or until onions are very soft. Add thyme, vinegar and honey and cook, uncovered, another 5 minutes until onions are caramelised.

Toss zucchini with 1 teaspoon sea salt and stand for 30 minutes. Cook beans in simmering salted water about 2 minutes or until tender. Drain, rinse under cold water, then cut into 1 cm pieces.

Combine zucchini, beans, spinach, tofu, herbs, eggs, and 35 g (1/4 cup) of the sesame seeds, mix well and season to taste. Spoon vegetable mixture into a lightly greased and base-lined 24 cm springform pan, smooth top with a spatula and sprinkle with remaining sesame seeds. Bake at 180°C about 35 minutes or until set. Rest in pan for 10 minutes before removing to a plate.

Serve wedges of frittata with Braised Onions and Leafy Green Salad.

SERVES 6–8

Recipe can be made a day ahead.
Will keep, covered, in refrigerator.

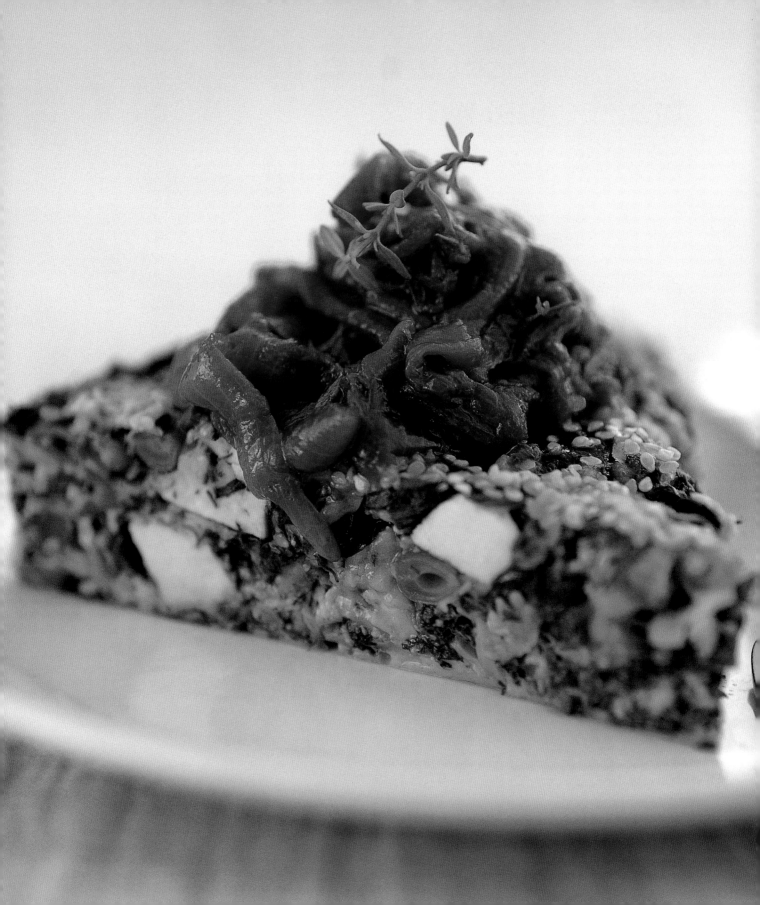

braised tofu with shiitake mushrooms

While tofu is quite bland in itself, it is a wonderful carrier of flavours and is one of our favourite ingredients. Jan has always cooked with it extensively, while Kathy is a recent convert.

1 tbsp soy sauce or wheat-free tamari sauce

1 tsp sesame oil

270 g firm tofu, cut into 12 pieces

25 g dried shiitake mushrooms soaked in 250 ml (1 cup) hot water for 30 minutes

200 ml Vegetable Stock (page 159)

light olive oil

6 green (spring) onions, sliced

3 cm piece ginger, thinly sliced

3 cloves garlic, chopped

1 large carrot, sliced thinly on the diagonal

100 g snowpeas, trimmed

1 bunch Chinese broccoli, thick ends trimmed, and sliced into 3 crosswise

1 baby bok choy, trimmed and leaves separated

steamed basmati rice, cooked according to directions on packet, to serve

Chilli Sauce (page166), to serve

Combine soy sauce and sesame oil in a bowl, add tofu and toss gently. Stand at room temperature for 30 minutes.

Drain mushrooms and remove stalks, reserve soaking water and add to stock. Heat a wok, add 2 teaspoons oil, green onions, ginger and garlic and stir-fry over high heat for 1 minute. Add carrot and mushrooms and stir-fry another minute. Add tofu mixture and stock, bring to the boil and simmer gently, covered, for 5 minutes. Add snowpeas and simmer, uncovered, another 3 minutes. Remove mixture from wok and keep warm.

Heat 2 teaspoons oil in same wok and stir-fry Chinese broccoli and bok choy over high heat until just wilted.

Place greens in the base of shallow bowls and spoon tofu mixture and braising liquid over. Serve with steamed rice and Chilli Sauce.

SERVES 4

Recipe best made just before serving.

menus for special occasions

*We are suggesting these two menus for a special occasion when you want to lash out and entertain.
Go to town and have some fun in the kitchen. Your guests will love the clean fresh flavours and will
never know you are detoxing.*

SUMMER MENU

Tamari Nuts	36
Seared Tuna & Asparagus Salad with Tamari Dressing	74
Chargrilled Lamb Backstrap with Caper & Olive Salsa	104
Poached Peaches with Maple Syrup & Yoghurt	154

WINTER MENU

Spice, Nut & Seed Dip with Vegetables	34
Pumpkin & Garlic Soup with Smoked Tofu	48
Baked Snapper with Braised Fennel & Leeks and Lentils	116
Warm Pears with Honey & Walnuts	149

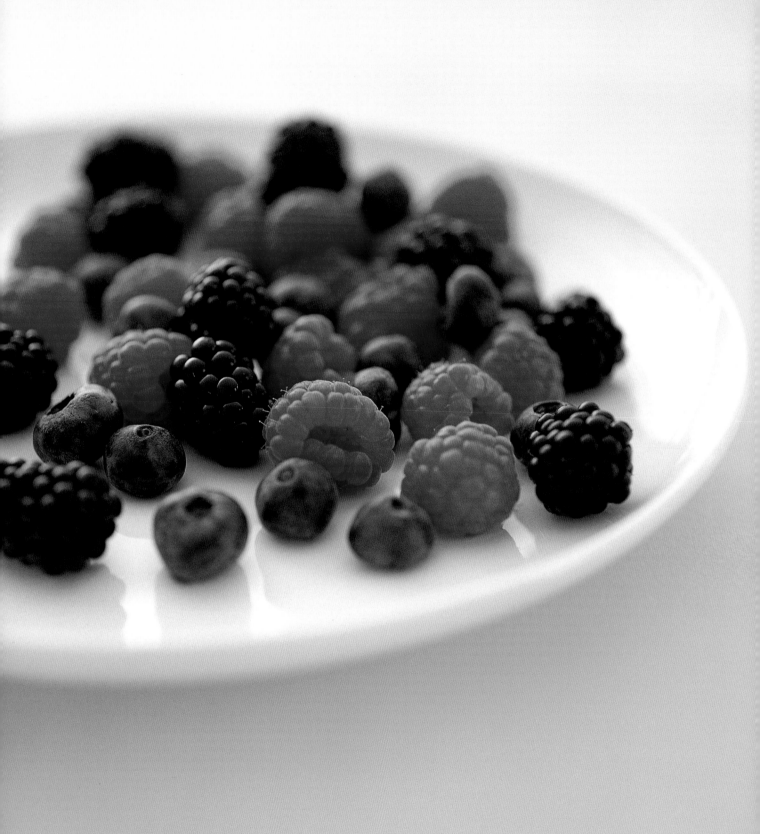

dessert

If you have a sweet tooth, one of the hardest things to avoid during a detox is dessert. Sugar is definitely off the list when detoxing, however, it is still possible to enjoy naturally sweet foods made into delightful combinations. We recommend that you don't have a dessert as such each day, but save them for two to three times per week. Instead of a 'proper' dessert, have a lovely piece of fresh fruit with some natural soy yoghurt if you're looking for extras after dinner. For dessert nights, try one of our ten great desserts – just the ticket when you're entertaining or enjoying a good dinner in.

If you are out to dinner and are not sure what you can eat on the menu, ask the waiter if you can have some fresh fruit. Many restaurants will accommodate such a simple request, providing they actually serve fresh fruit with desserts on the menu. If they serve a cheese plate with dried fruit and nuts, you could ask for that – without the cheese of course. Otherwise, it may be best to abstain and enjoy one of your own desserts as part of another meal at home.

We use natural rice syrup, honey and maple syrup as the main sweeteners in our dessert recipes. However, we also use sweet fresh fruit or dried fruit to achieve the most satisfying flavour.

warm poached dried fruit with rosewater

This makes a fruity rich dessert and because the fruit is high in natural sugar, there is no need for sweetening. You can serve the fruit with the Almond Cream (page 157) or it teams well with the Pistachio, Honey & Cardamom Ice-Cream (page 153). Use preservative-free dried fruit.

4 dried figs, stems removed

35 g (¼ cup) raisins

2 tbsp sultanas

8 prunes

4 dried apricots

¼ tsp ground mace

½ vanilla bean, split lengthways

2–3 tsp rosewater, to taste

Combine figs, raisins, sultanas, prunes, apricots and mace with 250 ml (1 cup) water in a saucepan. Use small sharp knife to scrape vanilla seeds from pod into pan. Add pod to pan. Bring to a simmer over medium heat. Reduce to low and cook gently, covered, stirring occasionally, for 20 minutes or until fruit is soft but retains its shape. Remove from heat, gently stir in rosewater to taste and allow to cool until warm. Remove and discard the vanilla pod.

Spoon poached fruit into bowls to serve.

SERVES 4

Fruit can be poached a day ahead and kept, covered, in refrigerator. Warm before serving if you like.

indian spiced rice pudding with sultanas & almonds

The sultanas in this pudding make a lovely addition without the need for additional sweetening. We love the Indian spices because they add to the flavour, creating their own fragrant sweetness.

110 g (¹/₂ cup) medium-grain rice

1 L (4 cups) rice milk or reduced-fat soy milk

45 g (¹/₄ cup) sultanas

1 cinnamon stick

¹/₂ vanilla bean, split lengthways

5 cardamom pods, lightly crushed

¹/₄ tsp ground nutmeg

40 g (¹/₄ cup) slivered almonds, toasted

Place rice, rice milk or soy milk, sultanas, cinnamon, vanilla, cardamom and nutmeg in a saucepan and bring to a simmer over medium heat. Reduce heat and cook gently, partially covered, stirring often, for 1 to 1¹/₄ hours or until rice is very soft and mixture has a porridge consistency.

Stir in half the almonds. Spoon into dishes and sprinkle with remaining almonds. Serve warm or at room temperature.

SERVES 4

Pudding will keep for 2 days in an airtight container in refrigerator. Warm before serving if using. Add almonds just before serving.

grilled mango cheeks with lime & coconut ice

A light and delicious dessert – perfect for a hot summer's day. To make the ice easier to scoop, pop it in the refrigerator for 10 minutes or so to soften slightly. If you prefer, serve the mango fresh without grilling.

2 large ripe mangoes

2 tsp of maple syrup

lime rind strips to serve

LIME & COCONUT ICE

1 x 400 ml can light coconut milk

160 ml (2/3 cup) apple and peach juice
  (no added sugar)

finely grated rind and juice of 1 lime

1 1/2 tbsp maple syrup

To make Lime & Coconut Ice, combine coconut milk, apple and peach juice, lime rind, lime juice and maple syrup in a bowl. Mix well. Pour into a non-aluminium freezer-proof container and freeze, stirring with a fork occasionally to break up the ice crystals, for 6 hours or until just frozen through. Use a hand blender to process until smooth. Alternatively, scoop into the bowl of a food processor and process until smooth. Return to freezer container. Cover and freeze for a further 2 hours or until firm.

Cut cheeks from mangoes and score flesh into diamonds. Brush with maple syrup and place, cut-side up on oven tray. Cook under a hot grill (or place cut-side down on preheated chargrill pan) for 2 minutes or until lightly browned and fragrant. Place mango on flat serving plates. Scoop lime and coconut ice into small bowls and sprinkle with lime rind strips. Place on serving plates beside mango and serve immediately.

SERVES 4

You can make the Lime & Coconut Ice up to 2 weeks ahead, and keep, tightly covered, in freezer. Grill or chargrill the mango just before serving.

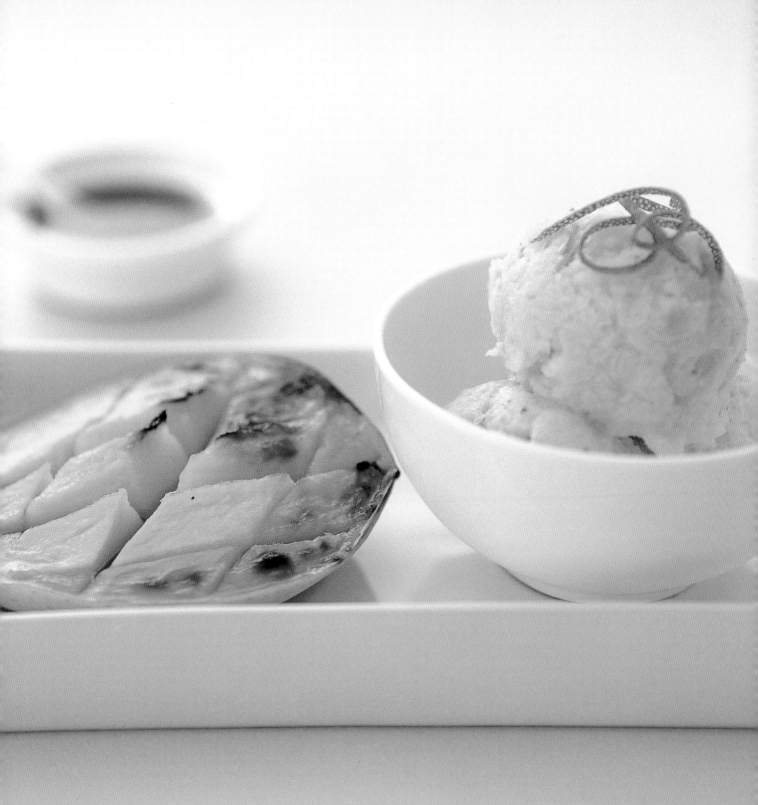

apple & berry crumble

If you're like Jan, you enjoy a good fruit crumble for dessert on a cool night. This is a lovely crumble because the apples are lightly stewed to bring out their flavour. Use thawed frozen berries if fresh ones are not available. You can also make this in individual 1-cup ovenproof dishes.

4 red apples, peeled, cored and
    quartered
300 g berries (such as strawberries,
    raspberries, blackberries or
    blueberries)
1 tsp honey
light olive oil for greasing

TOPPING
125 g (1^{1}/3 cups) rolled oats
35 g (^{1}/3 cup) rice bran
^{1}/2 tsp ground cinnamon
^{1}/2 tsp freshly grated or ground nutmeg
^{1}/4 tsp allspice
1 tbsp macadamia or canola oil
2 tsp butter, melted
3 tsp honey

To make filling, place apples in saucepan and add 180 ml (^{3}/4 cup) water. Bring to a simmer and cook, covered, for 10 minutes or until just tender. Drain off the liquid and add berries and honey. Mix gently.

Lightly brush a shallow 2-litre (8-cup) ovenproof dish with oil. Place apple mixture in dish.

To make Topping, combine oats, rice bran, cinnamon, nutmeg and allspice in a bowl. Mix well. Combine oil, butter and honey, and pour over oat mixture. Use your fingers to rub the mixture together to evenly combine. Sprinkle mixture over apples. Bake at 180°C for 15 minutes or until topping is lightly browned. Serve warm or at room temperature.

SERVES 4–6

Crumble can be made several hours ahead
and baked just before serving.

warm pears with honey & walnuts

This is a twist on a traditional baked apple recipe. Instead, we use pears, sultanas and dates to give delicious natural sweetness. You can also use apple halves if you like.

2 tbsp toasted and chopped walnuts

2 tbsp chopped dried dates

2 tbsp sultanas

3 tsp honey

2 tsp butter, melted

4 pears, halved, cored and peeled

Almond Cream (page 157), to serve

Combine walnuts, dates and sultanas in a bowl. Combine honey, butter and 2 tablespoons water in a small jug. Place pears in shallow ovenproof dish in a single layer. Spoon walnut mixture onto each pear then drizzle honey mixture over the top. Cover dish with foil and bake at 180°C for 30 minutes or until pears are tender. Serve warm or at room temperature with a drizzle of Almond Cream.

SERVES 4

Pears can be baked several hours ahead.

grapefruit salad with toasted macadamias & almond cream

While oranges are on the 'avoid' list, you can still enjoy grapefruit in season. You may prefer to use all pink grapefruit, or a mixture of pink and yellow as we have here.

45 g (¼ cup) unsalted macadamia nuts

1 pink grapefruit

1 yellow grapefruit

1 tbsp brown rice syrup

1 tsp orange blossom water

Almond Cream (page 157)

Spread nuts on oven tray and roast at 180°C for 5 minutes or until golden. Cool 10 minutes then coarsely chop. Set aside.

Use a zester to remove coloured skin from the pink grapefruit (or use a vegetable peeler to thinly remove the rind avoiding white pith, then cut the rind into thin strips). Peel both grapefruit, removing all white pith. Use a sharp knife to cut between membranes and remove segments, holding fruit over bowl to catch juices.

Combine zest, segments and any juice in bowl with rice syrup and orange blossom water. Gently stir until combined, then stir in nuts. Set aside to macerate for 20 minutes.

Spoon into bowls and serve accompanied by Almond Cream.

SERVES 4

Salad will keep for 6 hours, covered, in refrigerator.

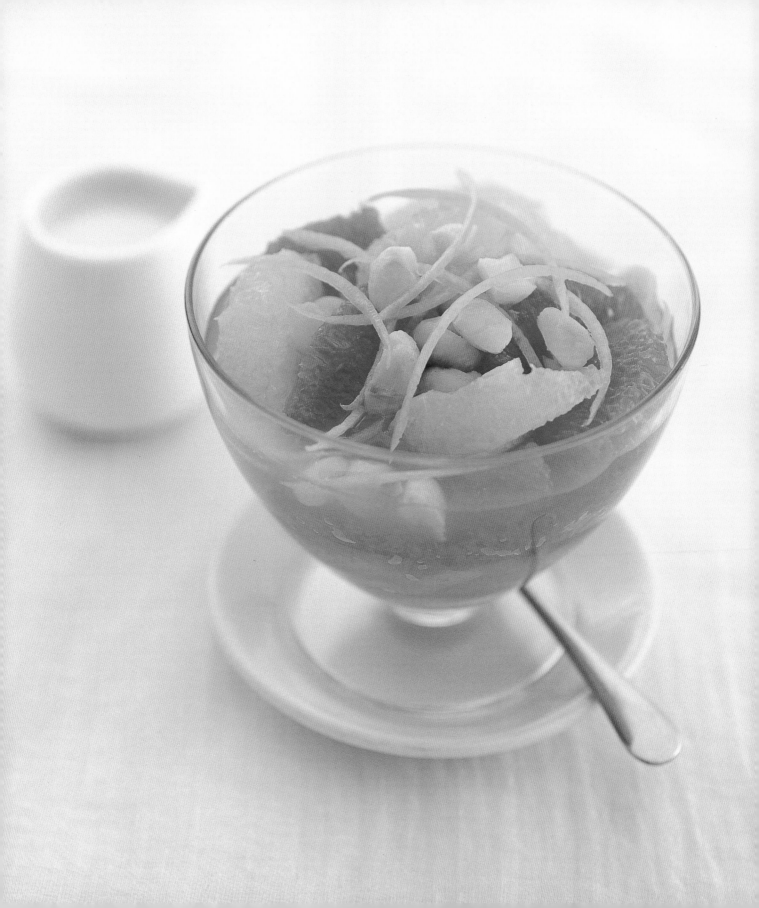

baked fruit parcels
with passionfruit

We've used fabulous summer fruit in this recipe, however, you can use fruit in season at any time of year. For example, a winter combination could be apple, pear, custard apple, tamarillo, banana and passionfruit.

2 nectarines, halved and stones
 removed

2 plums or peaches, halved and stones
 removed

1 mango, cheeks removed, peeled and
 sliced

1 banana, peeled and sliced on the
 diagonal

12 cherries or strawberries, stems
 removed

20 g (¼ cup) shredded coconut, toasted

2 tsp honey

2 passionfruit

Cut 4 x 30 cm lengths of baking paper. Place paper on bench. Divide fruit onto centre of paper and sprinkle with coconut. Drizzle with honey and passionfruit pulp. Fold paper to enclose fruit and create parcels. Place parcels on oven tray.

Bake at 180°C for 15 minutes or until fruit is heated and steaming. Place parcels on serving plates and cool for 3 minutes before serving.

SERVES 4

Parcels can be assembled 1 hour ahead
then baked close to serving.

pistachio, honey & cardamom ice-cream

This ice-cream has a refreshing icy consistency and teams really well with sweet fresh fruit such as Bethonga pineapple, banana, ripe stone fruit and fresh figs. If you're not fond of cardamom, use ground cinnamon instead. To make the ice-cream easier to scoop, place it in the refrigerator for 10 minutes or so to soften slightly.

500 ml (2 cups) reduced fat soy milk

400 g (2 cups) plain soy yoghurt

2 tbsp honey

³/₄ tsp ground cardamom

75 g (¹/₂ cup) shelled pistachio nuts

fresh fruit slices, to serve

Place soy milk, yoghurt, honey and cardamom in a bowl and whisk until well combined. Pour into a non-aluminium freezer-proof container, cover and freeze for 6 hours or until just frozen through.

Meanwhile, soak pistachio nuts in hot water for 20 minutes. Peel off the skins and coarsely chop nuts.

Use a hand blender to puree ice-cream until smooth. Alternatively, scoop into the bowl of a food processor and process until smooth. Place in airtight container and stir in chopped nuts. Cover and freeze for 2 hours or until firm.

Serve a scoop or two of ice-cream with fruit.

SERVES 6–8

Ice-cream will keep for up to 2 weeks in an airtight container in freezer.

poached peaches with maple syrup & yoghurt

Peaches in season are pure perfection. Lightly poaching them enhances their colour and makes them easy to eat with a spoon. Choose peaches with rich colour. You can also use nectarines in this recipe. The peaches also work well with Lime & Coconut Ice (page 146) or the Pistachio, Honey & Cardamom Ice-Cream (page 153).

1 cinnamon stick, broken into pieces

1 vanilla bean, split lengthways

4 large, well-coloured, ripe peaches

1 tbsp pure maple syrup

vanilla soy yoghurt, to serve (optional)

Combine 750 ml (3 cups) water, cinnamon and vanilla in a large saucepan. Bring to the boil and cook, covered, for 5 minutes. Reduce to a gentle simmer. Use a small sharp knife to cut just through the skin along the natural seam in the peaches. Add peaches to the pan and cook, covered, turning once or twice, for 4–5 minutes or until a skewer inserts into the flesh easily. Use a slotted spoon to place peaches on a plate. Boil the liquid, uncovered, for 5 minutes.

Use a small sharp knife to peel away peach skins and place peaches in a bowl. Combine 2 tablespoons of the cooking liquid with the maple syrup and pour over peaches.

Serve peaches with yoghurt, if using.

SERVES 4

Peaches can be poached up to 2 days ahead. Keep, covered, in refrigerator. Bring to room temperature before serving.

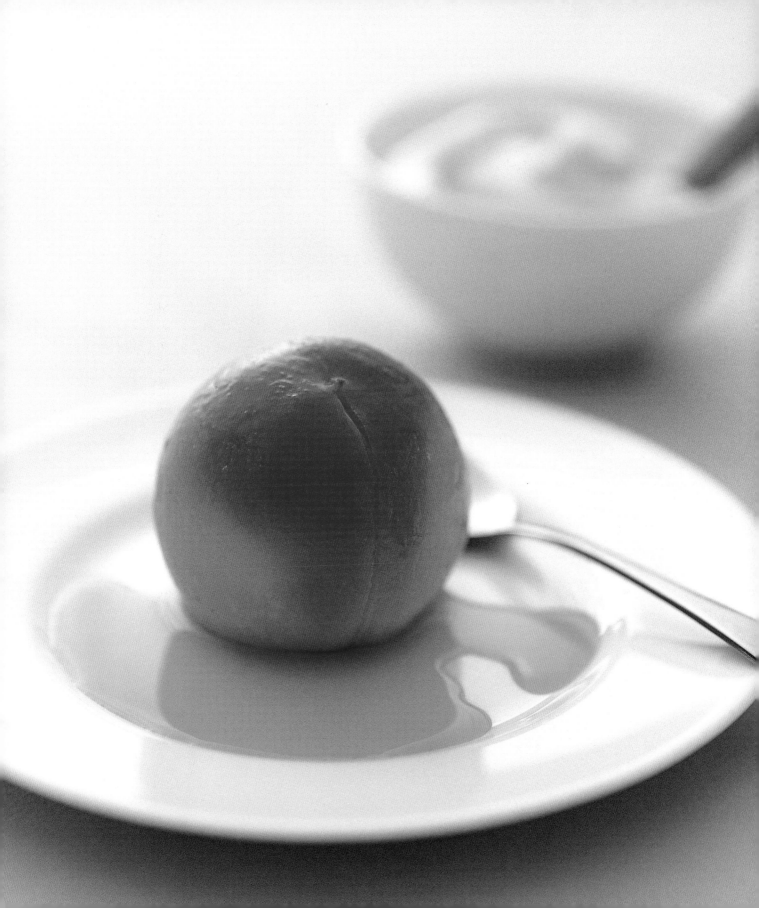

baked rice & rhubarb custards

A favourite good old fashioned comfort food is baked rice custard. Jan's nana used to make an excellent one. Rather than going without when detoxing, we came up with this version. You can use soy milk for a creamier taste if you prefer.

75 g (1/3 cup) medium-grain rice

vegetable or canola oil

3 stalks (about 160 g) rhubarb, cut into
   2 cm lengths

2 eggs

1 egg white

500 ml (2 cups) rice milk

1 x 140 g container apple fruit puree

1 tbsp honey

1 tsp pure vanilla essence

1/2 tsp ground nutmeg

Cook rice following packet directions until tender. Drain. Lightly brush 4 x 250 ml (1 cup) ovenproof dishes with vegetable or canola oil. Place rhubarb and rice into dishes. Place dishes in a roasting pan.

Whisk eggs, egg white, rice milk, apple puree, honey, vanilla and nutmeg in a large jug until well combined. Carefully pour into dishes.

Pour enough boiling water into roasting pan to come halfway up side of dishes. Bake at 180° for 40 minutes or until a knife inserted in the centres comes out clean. Remove dishes from water bath and serve warm or at room temperature.

SERVES 4

Puddings are best eaten on day of cooking, but they will keep quite well, covered, in refrigerator for 1 day.

almond cream

This is a substitute for thickened cream and teams particularly well with fruit desserts. You can flavour the cream with finely grated orange, lime or lemon rind and use a little of the citrus juice in place of the same quantity of water. Here we keep the flavour quite neutral to make it a good all-rounder recipe. Unlike regular dairy cream, this cream is a good source of dietary fibre as well as calcium.

185 ml (3/4 cup) water
150 g (1 1/2 cups) almond meal
95 g (1/2 cup) plain soy yoghurt
1 tbsp honey

Place water, almond meal, yoghurt and honey in a jug and use a hand blender to mix until the consistency of thickened pouring cream. Alternatively, place in a blender jug and blend until well combined.

MAKES ABOUT 2 CUPS

Cream will keep for up to 3 days in an airtight container in refrigerator.

basics

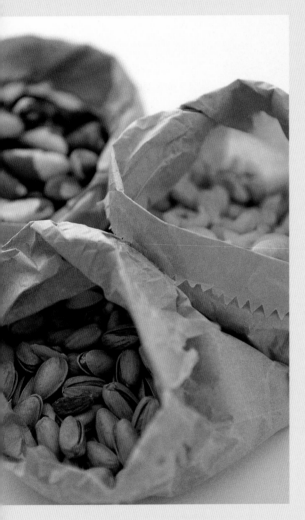

These recipes either appear frequently in the cookbook, or are recipes that you might use on a regular day-to-day basis, such as The Big Salad (see page 163), one of our favourite stand-bys or Hummus (see page 165) which is great to pack for snacks with rice crackers or have as part of your lunch.

We make stock on a weekly basis so it's always on hand for a soup or a sauce or risotto. It is really important to simmer stock at a low temperature and to skim it regularly. This will give you a lovely clear stock instead of a cloudy and murky result. If you need to remove the fat from the surface of chicken stock before it has had time to cool and solidify, simply run a sheet of plastic wrap over the surface of the stock and it will collect the fat.

If you want to freeze stock, allow it to cool before placing in airtight containers in the freezer. To take up less space in the freezer you can reduce chicken and vegetable stock (not fish stock). After straining the stock, boil, uncovered, over high heat until reduced by two-thirds. Then cool and pack in airtight containers. Once thawed, you can add water to reconstitute it before you use it.

chicken stock

For some useful tips about making this stock, see page 158.

1 kg chicken wings, rinsed

1 carrot, coarsely chopped

1 stick celery, coarsely chopped

1 onion, halved

6 stalks fresh parsley

4 sprigs fresh thyme

1 fresh or dried bay leaf

6 black peppercorns

Combine all ingredients in a large stockpot, add 3 litres (12 cups) water and bring slowly to the boil, skimming scum as it rises to the surface. Reduce heat to a gentle simmer and cook, uncovered, for 2 hours, adding more water if necessary. Strain stock through a sieve lined with a muslin cloth and discard solids. Cool, cover and refrigerate until cold, then remove fat from surface.

MAKES ABOUT 2 LITRES (8 CUPS)

Will keep, covered, in refrigerator for 3 days or can be reduced and frozen for 1 month.

vegetable stock

Almost any vegetables can go into this stock, depending on what is at hand, including spinach. If you do add spinach, just remember you will get a murky looking stock instead of a clear result.

2 onions, quartered

2 carrots, chopped

3 tomatoes, chopped

1 tbsp olive oil

2 sticks celery, chopped

4 mushrooms, sliced

1 fresh or dried bay leaf

6 black peppercorns

Combine onions, carrots and tomatoes in a large roasting pan and toss with oil. Roast at 200°C for 30 minutes or until browned. Transfer vegetables to a large stockpot, add remaining ingredients and cover with 3 litres (12 cups) water. Bring to the boil, skimming scum as it rises to the surface. Reduce heat and simmer, uncovered, for 2 hours. Strain stock through a muslin-lined sieve and discard solids. Cool, cover and refrigerate until ready to use.

MAKES ABOUT 2 LITRES (8 CUPS)

Will keep, covered, in the refrigerator for 4 days or can be frozen for 1 month.

fish stock

Once fish stock has come to the boil, it is essential that you simmer it for no longer than 30 minutes or it will develop a bitter flavour. Chop the vegetables finely to extract maximum flavour in the short cooking time.

fish bones (the frame and head of a blue
  eye or snapper or other white fish)

2 carrots, finely chopped

2 sticks celery, finely chopped

1 onion, quartered

3 tomatoes, chopped

6 stalks fresh parsley

6 sprigs fresh thyme

1 fresh or dried bay leaf

6 black peppercorns

Combine all ingredients in a large stockpot, add 3 litres (12 cups) water and bring slowly to the boil, skimming scum as it rises to the surface. Reduce heat to a gentle simmer and cook, uncovered, for 30 minutes. Strain stock through a sieve lined with a muslin cloth and discard solids. When stock has cooled, strain again, leaving any sediment behind. Cool, cover and refrigerate until ready to use.

MAKES ABOUT 2.5 LITRES (10 CUPS)

Will keep, covered, in refrigerator for 3 days or can be frozen for 1 month.

garlic mash

Mash is such wonderful comfort food, and it's reassuring to know you can still eat it while you are detoxing. Here we substitute soy milk and stock for butter and cow's milk. It gives a lighter result. Leave the garlic out if you wish.

600 g potatoes, peeled and cut into
  pieces

600 ml Chicken or Vegetable Stock
  (page 159)

2 cloves garlic, crushed

60 ml (1/4 cup) soy milk

Cover potatoes with stock and bring to the boil, then simmer, uncovered, over low heat until tender. Strain and reserve stock.

Mash potatoes with garlic, soy milk and 60 ml (1/4 cup) of the warm stock until smooth, adding more stock if necessary.

SERVES 4

Mash best made close to serving.

poached chicken

Delicious tossed with lots of crisp green salad leaves, avocado, finely chopped celery, a few spoons of Light Mayonnaise (page 164) and some tarragon leaves. The added bonus of poaching a whole chicken is that you also have the stock. If you like, you can simmer stock over high heat and reduce by half to intensify the flavour before you strain it.

1.8 kg chicken, rinsed

1 onion, halved

1 leek, coarsely chopped

1 large carrot, chopped

1 large stick celery, chopped

4 stalks fresh parsley

4 sprigs fresh thyme

1 fresh or dried bay leaf

6 black peppercorns

Combine chicken and remaining ingredients in a large stockpot and add enough cold water to cover by 2 cm. Bring slowly to the boil, skimming scum as it rises to the surface. Reduce heat to a gentle simmer and cook, partially covered, for 45 minutes. Cool chicken in stock for 30 minutes, then remove from pot. Strain stock through a sieve lined with a damp muslin cloth and discard solids. Cool, cover and refrigerate until cold, then remove fat from surface. Chicken can be used in salads, tossed with rice noodles, or added to a soup.

MAKES ABOUT 3 LITRES (12 CUPS) STOCK

Stock and chicken will keep, covered, in the refrigerator for 3 days. Stock can be reduced and frozen for 1 month.

leafy green salad

We love a leafy salad, made with soft leaves that can go with just about anything. Lots of green leaves is our mantra when detoxing. You can vary the flavour of the dressing depending on what you are serving it with, and add other ingredients such as tomatoes, asparagus, cucumbers and toasted nuts and seeds.

150 g mixed soft salad leaves, including
   butter lettuce, oak leaf, mignonette,
   watercress sprigs or radicchio, torn
   into bite-sized pieces

1 tbsp extra virgin olive oil

2 tsp lemon juice, balsamic vinegar or
   verjuice

Toss leaves with oil and juice, vinegar or verjuice and season to taste.

SERVES 4 AS AN ACCOMPANIMENT

Salad best made just before serving.

baby spinach salad

You could add some chunks of tofu and blanched asparagus or poached chicken to this salad to make it a main course.
If you suffer from migraines, you could substitute segmented grapefruit for the oranges (oranges are a common trigger).

150 g baby spinach

2 tsp soy sauce, wheat-free tamari or
   balsamic vinegar

1 tbsp extra virgin olive oil

1/2 avocado, seeded, peeled and sliced

1 orange, peeled and segmented

20 g (1/4 cup) flaked almonds, toasted

Toss spinach with soy sauce, tamari or balsamic vinegar and olive oil and season to taste. Place in a salad bowl and top with avocado, orange and almonds.

SERVES 4 AS AN ACCOMPANIMENT

Salad best made just before serving.

roasted beetroot & rocket salad

This is another simple salad using one of our favourite ingredients, roasted beetroot. We are in the habit of roasting a bunch of beetroot on a weekly basis and keeping it in the refrigerator to use whenever. Roasting beetroot in foil keeps in all the flavour and goodness and makes them really easy to peel. You can add more vegetables such as roasted sweet potato to this salad to make it more substantial.

2 large beetroot, trimmed

150 g baby rocket

1 tbsp extra virgin olive oil

2 tsp red wine vinegar

1/2 avocado, seeded, peeled and cut into
   2 cm pieces

30 g (1/4 cup) walnuts, toasted

1 tbsp chopped fresh chives

Wrap beetroot in foil, place on an oven tray and roast at 200°C for 50–60 minutes until tender. Remove foil and, when cool enough to handle, peel away skins and cut into wedges.

Toss rocket with oil and vinegar and season to taste. Place in a salad bowl and top with avocado, beetroot, walnuts and chives.

SERVES 4 AS AN ACCOMPANIMENT

Roasted beetroot will keep, covered, in refrigerator for 3 days.
Salad best made just before serving.

the big salad

Serve as an accompaniment or, if you want to make it a substantial meal, serve with hummus, or toss in some poached chicken, chargrilled lamb, tuna or salmon. You can add what you like – roasted vegetables, some fresh herbs and a wedge of avocado. Verjuice is the juice of unfermented ripe grapes and is lovely added to sauces and used in dressings. You can buy it in good delis.

2 egg (Roma) tomatoes, halved
   lengthwise
100 g small Swiss brown mushrooms
extra virgin olive oil
150 g mixed leaves (can include rocket,
   mesclun, cos or baby spinach)
1 tbsp lemon juice, verjuice, white wine
   vinegar, red wine vinegar or balsamic
   vinegar
roasted vegetables of your choice, such as
   wedges of pumpkin
1 small Lebanese (small green)
   cucumber, cut into wedges
1 avocado, peeled, seeded and quartered
1/4 cup fresh basil leaves

Place tomatoes and mushrooms on an oven tray, brush lightly with olive oil and season to taste. Roast at 150°C for 30 minutes.

Toss leaves with 1 tablespoon olive oil and lemon juice, verjuice or vinegar and top with tomatoes, mushrooms, roasted vegetables, cucumber and avocado, then sprinkle with basil leaves.

SERVES 4

Salad best made just before serving.

roasted capsicum

Roasting capsicum really intensifies their flavour. Make sure to collect all the juices when you are peeling and seeding them, as they form their own dressing.

2 red capsicums

Place capsicums on an oven tray and roast at 200°C for 30 minutes, turning occasionally, or until skins are blistered and blackened.

Remove from oven and cover loosely with foil on tray for 10 minutes. When cool enough to handle, peel and seed capsicum and cut into 2 cm-wide strips. Mix with their juices.

Will keep, covered, in refrigerator for 3 days.

yoghurt dressing

A simple dressing for grilled fish, lamb or grilled vegetables. As a guide, use dill, chives and coriander to go with fish; and tarragon, basil and mint to go with chicken; and basil, coriander and parsley to go with lamb.

200 g plain soy yoghurt

2 cloves garlic, crushed

2 tbsp chopped fresh mixed herbs

2 tbsp lemon juice

1 tbsp extra virgin olive oil

1/2 tsp Dijon mustard

Combine all ingredients, whisk together and season to taste. Stand for 30 minutes for flavours to develop.

MAKES ABOUT 1 CUP

Will keep, covered, in refrigerator for 3 days.

tahini dressing

This dressing is suitable to toss with salad leaves, or to drizzle over roasted vegetables, grilled fish or lamb.

60 ml (1/4 cup) tahini

2 cloves garlic, crushed

2 tbsp lemon juice

1 tbsp extra virgin olive oil

Combine all ingredients, whisk in 60 ml (1/4 cup) water and season to taste. Stand for 30 minutes for flavours to develop.

MAKES ABOUT 1 CUP

Will keep, covered, in refrigerator for 1 week.

light mayonnaise

Because of the small quantity you are dealing with here, you need to use a mini food processor or hand-held blender or make this mayonnaise by hand with a balloon whisk – this quantity would be lost in the bowl of a regular food processor.

1 egg yolk

1 clove garlic, chopped

1 tbsp lemon juice

1/2 tsp Dijon mustard

100 ml olive oil

Combine egg yolk, garlic, juice and mustard in a small hand-held blender and process until smooth. Add oil slowly in a thin stream and process until thick. Add 1–2 tablespoons water and process until smooth. Season to taste.

MAKES ABOUT 200 ML

Will keep, covered, in the refrigerator for 3 days.

hummus

You can make hummus with canned chickpeas, but it is so much nicer made with the dried variety, or you can buy it ready-made from supermarkets or good food stores. It's a great accompaniment to a plate of roasted vegetables or as an accompaniment to The Big Salad (page 163). It's also good with crudités or spread on rye toast and topped with roasted tomatoes, or served with our Spiced Bran Crackers (page 35).

200 g (1 cup) dried chickpeas, soaked
  in cold water overnight

2 dried bay leaves

1/2 onion

2 cloves garlic, chopped

125 ml (1/2 cup) lemon juice

60 ml (1/4 cup) tahini

Sweet paprika and extra virgin
  olive oil, to serve

Cook drained chickpeas, bay leaves and onion, uncovered, in simmering water about 30 minutes or until chickpeas are tender. Drain, reserve cooking liquid and discard bay leaves and onion.

Combine chickpeas and remaining ingredients in a food processor and process until smooth, adding 100–150 ml cooking liquid, to form a smooth paste. Season to taste.

Serve sprinkled with sweet paprika and drizzled with a little olive oil.

MAKES ABOUT 2 1/2 CUPS

Will keep, covered, in refrigerator for 5 days.

tahini & almond spread

An excellent base for spelt or rye bruschetta which can be topped with chopped tomato or roasted pumpkin, red onion and avocado. Also suitable as a dip with crudités.

125 g blanched almonds

60 ml (1/4 cup) tahini

2 tbsp lemon juice

Place almonds on an oven tray and roast at 200°C for 5–10 minutes or until golden. Cool.

Process almonds, tahini, lemon juice and 125 ml (1/2 cup) water until a smooth paste forms. Season to taste.

MAKES ABOUT 1 1/4 CUPS

Spread will keep, covered, in refrigerator for 2 weeks.

chilli sauce

This is a good standby chilli sauce and can be used with a number of dishes such as the Spicy Blue Eye & Green Pawpaw Stir-Fry (page 68). The addition of a little maple syrup or honey gives balance to the heat of the chillies. The heat of the sauce will vary with the heat of the chillies – the older the chillies the hotter they will be. If it is too hot, add a little water to thin it down.

6 large fresh red chillies, chopped

juice of 2–3 limes, to taste

3 cloves garlic, chopped

1/4 tsp pure maple syrup or honey

sea salt

Combine all ingredients in the small bowl of a food processor and process until smooth. Season to taste with sea salt.

MAKES ABOUT 1/2 CUP

Will keep, covered, in refrigerator for 4 days.

dukkah

Dukkah is a delicious Mediterranean spice mix that is traditionally served with a dish of olive oil and bread for dipping. Don't overprocess the dukkah in the spice grinder or you will end up with a paste rather than a dry spice mix.

1 tbsp cumin seeds

1 tbsp coriander seeds

20 g hazelnuts

20 g blanched almonds

2 tbsp sesame seeds

Dry roast cumin and coriander seeds in a frying pan over low heat until fragrant. Cool.

Combine cumin and coriander seeds in a spice grinder and process until ground. Transfer ground spices to the bowl of a small food processor, add nuts and process until just smooth. Stir in sesame seeds and season to taste.

MAKES ABOUT 2/3 CUP DUKKAH

Dukkah will keep in an airtight container for 1 month